800

THE PAP SMEAR

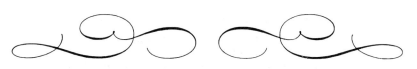

THE PAP SMEAR

Life of

George N. Papanicolaou

By

D. Erskine Carmichael, M.D.

Clinical Associate Professor of Obstetrics and Gynecology
University of Alabama in Birmingham
The Medical Center
Birmingham, Alabama

With a Foreword by

Charles S. Cameron, M.D.

Chairman of the Board, Hahnemann Medical College and Hospital
Philadelphia, Pennsylvania

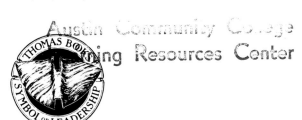

CHARLES C THOMAS • PUBLISHER

Springfield · Illinois · U.S.A.

Published and Distributed Throughout the World by

CHARLES C THOMAS • PUBLISHER

Bannerstone House

301-327 East Lawrence Avenue, Springfield, Illinois, U.S.A.

©*1973, by* CHARLES C THOMAS • PUBLISHER

ISBN 0-398-02716-1

Library of Congress Catalog Card Number: 72-93204

*With THOMAS BOOKS careful attention is given to all details of
manufacturing and design. It is the Publisher's desire to present books that are
satisfactory as to their physical qualities and artistic possibilities and
appropriate for their particular use. THOMAS BOOKS will be true to those
laws of quality that assure a good name and good will.*

Printed in the United States of America

R-1

This book is dedicated to
MRS. MARY G. PAPANICOLAOU
with admiration and affection

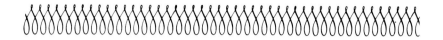

FOREWORD

IN the keynote remarks opening the World Conference on Cancer of the Uterus, conducted by the American Cancer Society in March 1969, I said " the two most striking changes which appear in current epidemiologic studies of cancer are the increase in death and incidence rates of cancer of the lung and the decrease in death rates of cancer of the uterus." Later, in concluding the address, I offered it as my belief "that the application of the exfoliative cytologic method (Papanicolaou test) to the detection of cancer and pre-cancer in the uterus has provided the chief single reason for the reduction of deaths from cancer of the uterus during the past twenty years. It has served to do so directly, and by the nature of its hopeful newness it has done so indirectly by stimulating professional and public enthusiasm.

It was among my life's greatest privileges to have known Dr. Papanicolaou from 1947 until his death in 1962. During these fifteen years our acquaintance ripened into a firm and warm friendship. As time went on, we found it helpful to meet rather regularly, he, to discuss his ambition to broaden and intensify the work he had begun, and I, to seek his advice on how the Cancer Society should develop programs designed to make the benefits of the cytologic method of diagnosis known to the widest possible audience. It happened that the midpoint between our two institutions in New York City – the Cornell Medical College and the American Cancer Society Headquarters – was the Plaza Hotel. It was in the bar of that establishment where we conducted much of our business.

The facts of Papanicolaou's career have been carefully

researched and faithfully recorded by Dr. Carmichael, so that much of what I could say has been said much better in his book.

However, I am grateful for the opportunity to record my personal estimate of the man. The impression which overrides all others is that of his apparently unlimited capacity for work. After each arduous, full day in the laboratory at Cornell, there was dinner and sometimes a half hour of relaxation listening to music which he dearly loved, and then another four hour session began at his microscope. The midnight oil was usually seen burning in the windows of his study at the house in Douglaston. It was much the same on weekends, interrupted only by occasional Saturday or Sunday afternoon parties, primarily for his laboratory staff and the frequent visiting scientists from this country and abroad.

The next vision of the man was his humility. When I first knew him the famous monograph had been published three years before and it had established him as a major pathfinder, although it would be some years for his achievement to be universally acknowledged. He was invited to become a member of a number of faculties and hospital staffs of distinguished institutions from coast to coast and, indeed, in other countries. He received numerous distinguished awards here and abroad. He was repeatedly sought to give honor lectures. But he remained his humble self. It was a kind of humility which I have never encountered before nor since. He was not ingratiating in any way; it was a blend of dignity, courtesy and selflessness. He was at all times most graciously grateful for every citation of appreciation of his work.

However, the Grecian blood was there and I have seen him seethe at prejudice, preconception and premature judgement. Although a number of pathologists and gynecologists recognized at the outset the enormous importance of his work, he often felt frustrated by the reluctance of his profession in general to acknowledge its potentialities. He was in the company of those who were ahead of their time.

Fortunately, he lived to see his cytological test for cancer, not only in the uterus, but in the lung and other organs, recognized as "the most practically significant advance in the control of cancer in our time."

On reflecting on his life, as I often have, it has seemed to me that his career reaffirms better than any example I can think of the virtues of toil and discipline. His life is also a superb instance of the "American success story" – the impoverished unknown immigrant who becomes an heroic figure, honored throughout his adopted country and the world. Finally, the circumstances of his first recognition of cancer cells in secretions he was examining for another reason, is a major addition to the record of happy accidents of scientific discovery – the phenomenon of serendipity. Accident though it may have been, it was no accident that it was his prepared mind which caused him to surmise immediately the significance of what he saw.

I was with him when he died, the morning after a joyous, jubilant day in the company of old friends. It was a day when he appeared completely happy, and he might have been rejoicing the thought "This is what I have lived for," because a new life seemed to lie ahead, the realization of a lifetime – his own institute.

Great as he was I do not see how he could have achieved his full measure of greatness without the love, the unfailing encourage-ment and the total commitment to his comfort and happiness of his wife, Mary.

At the end, his work far from completed, he brooded about the time left to him. How satisfied he would be if he knew that his work is going on and that his successors are determined that his life giving contribution shall be univer-sally recognized and utilized as we had dared to hope in the Plaza Bar.

Dr. Carmichael's biography is worthy of its great subject. It will serve, I trust, to keep fresh the memory of George Papanicolaou who has so well deserved his place among medicine's immortals.

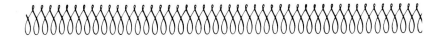

PREFACE

PROBABLY the most remarkable characteristic of George Papanicolaou was his strict mental and physical self-discipline. We find him developing this trait as a young boy as he forced himself to challange danger in order to overcome fear. Worried about his sentimentality as an expression of weakness, he was drawn to the German philosophy popular during his college days. It was the tremendous impact of the biophilosophy prevalent in Germany which urged him to forego any thought of medical practice and to continue his education with a study of the philosophical sciences. Initially captivated by the idealism so common to youth, he finally settled on a realistic, though ambitious, life goal in biological research.

A perfectionist in all details of life, Papanicolaou was patient in his striving and modest in his success, having faith, a sense of predestination that he would succeed. In addition to Pasteur's observation that " chance favors the prepared mind," Papanicolaou wondered "whether all our activities – scientific and otherwise – are actually governed by our own free will alone or also by forces lying beyond our grasp and control." In time, he was able to say that "one who has devoted his life's work to the furtherance of scientific knowledge may draw satisfaction from the conviction that he has within his own ability contributed to the enrichment of life and the alleviation of human suffering."

After success, he allowed himself many pleasures which he had to a great extent foregone in his zeal for his life's work. He reestablished ties with his family and indulged himself with music and the care of children. Even his scientific presentations began to expose his inner feeling for poetry as suggested in his description of his own role in the evolution of cytology: "It was at this stage of an apparent stalemate that a forceful movement made its appearance like a new tributary flowing into an old stream and helping it to gather new strength to surmount the obstacles which had blocked its further advancement."

Papanicolaou maintained his rather strict schedule for physical exercise throughout his life, swimming just several hours prior to his death at age seventy-eight years. It was his physical self which finally gave up; his mind was keen and perceptive to the end.

With a sense of humility for the privilege of looking intimately into the life of another and a sense of gratitude for the opportunity to accumulate some of the exciting facts surrounding this dedicated life, I submit the following biographical sketch of George N. Papanicolaou, a great man, a tower of strength.

D. ERSKINE CARMICHAEL

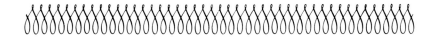

INTRODUCTION

IT is not often that a scientist who sets out to engage in pure research is able to witness universal acceptance and clinical application of his discoveries. Such was the case, however, of Dr. George Nicholas Papanicolaou. What began as zoological research involving the mechanism of sex determination resulted in a discovery "which in its significance in our fight against cancer stands unsurpassed in our century."* His research also enhanced the development of endocrinology during the third and fourth decades of this century to the extent that he has been called by one author "the father of modern endocrinology."† The contributions of Dr. Papanicolaou to the health and happiness of many thousands throughout the world represent the result of intellectual preparedness, determination and patience. To this must be added the dedication of a devoted wife who provided the support so critical to the exercise of these qualities in overcoming obstacles and disappointments common to such endeavors. Although he died at age seventy-eight just as he embarked on a new and promising scientific adventure, nevertheless George Papanicolaou had the satisfaction of knowing that his precepts originally considered of dubious value by his colleagues had become one of the cornerstones of diagnostic and preventive medicine and had established a new scientific discipline, cytology.

---

*Koss, Leopold G.: George N. Papanicolaou. *Acta Cytol,* 7(no. 3):145; 1963.
†Berkow, Samuel G.: After office hours – a visit with Dr. George N. Papanicolaou. *Obstet Gynecol, 16*(no. 2):248; 1960.

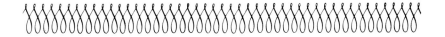

ACKNOWLEDGMENTS

ACCUMULATING and validating the biographical information contained in this monograph required the assistance and interest of many, most of whom were initially unknown to the author. To obtain details surrounding commonplace events which occurred in distant countries over half a century ago was often frustrating and occasionally impossible. It was indeed gratifying to learn the extent to which many kind friends and correspondents would pursue the difficult requests imposed on them.

Special thanks is given to Dr. S. Richardson Hill, Vice President of the University of Alabama in Birmingham, for his encouragement and assistance in this endeavor.

Mrs. George Papanicolaou, in her gracious and charming manner, made her reminiscences and memorabilia constantly available to me. My thanks to Dr. Charles Cameron, Chairman of the Board of Hahnemann Medical College and Hospital, for the use of his Papanicolaou biographical material, for his suggestions concerning the text, and for his Foreword. The American Cancer Society has generously provided funds for the publication of this work. All royalties have been assigned to this worthy organization for its continuing fight against the scourge of cancer.

Invaluable information was afforded by Mrs. Nina Stamatiou, sister of Dr. Papanicolaou, and Mrs. Maria Kokkoris, niece of the scientist. They provided a personal touch which would have been impossible to obtain elsewhere.

I am indebted to Dr. Basil Doumas, Dr. Maria Papaevangelos and Mrs. Maria Sepsas for their careful Greek translations, and to Mrs. Dominique Rust, formerly associated with the University of

Alabama Medical Center Library, for her detailed translation of the French.

Mr. Steve Papajohn enhanced the historical aspects of Kymi. Professor Karl von Frisch of Munich, and Professor O. Koehler of Freiburg, were faithful correspondents concerning the Papanicolaou years at the Hertwig Institute. Mme. J. Carpine-Lancre, of the Oceanographic Museum in Monaco, tirelessly answered my many inquiries.

Miss Charlotte Street; Mrs. J. F. Nonidez; Mrs. Grace Dickerson Wallace; Mrs. Herbert Traut; Dr. R. Gordon Douglas; Dr. Joseph Hinsey; Dr. Bernard Naylor; and the late Dr. Andrew Marchetti gave me special insight into the life of Dr. Papanicolaou after his arrival in the United States.

Without the selflessness, skill and patience of Miss L. Beatrice Ray, who typed and retyped the manuscript, the completion of this volume would not have been realized.

I am grateful for the many services provided for me by the University of Alabama Medical Center Library, under the direction of Mrs. Sarah Brown, and her able research librarian, Mrs. Hilda Harris; and to the staff of the Photography Department of the Medical Center who skillfully reproduced the photographs contained herein. Mr. Hugh Allman improved the quality of the photographs in Figures 6, 7, 11, 16, 17.

My appreciation should be expressed also to Dr. Masao Nakamoto for planting the seed of my inquiry into the life of Dr. Papanicolaou, and to Dr. Gene Ball for his review of the early chapters of the text.

My wife, Andrea, deserves special thanks for her cheerful acquiescence when evenings and vacations were required for the completion of the story.

D.E.C.

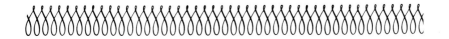

CONTENTS

THE PAP SMEAR

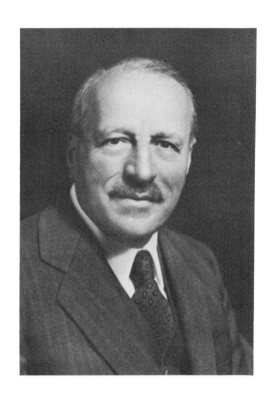

Figure 1.

George Nicholas Papanicolaou, Ph.D., M.D.
1883-1962

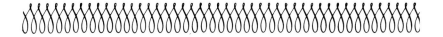

CHAPTER I

CHILDHOOD IN KYMI

LIFE was never severe for George Papanicolaou, for he spent his childhood in a picturesque seaport town, Kymi, on the eastern slopes of the Greek island, Euboea. His parents were upper middle class and they were committed to the proper intellectual and emotional development of their children.

Athanase Papanicolaou, grandfather of the scientist, had accumulated modest wealth during the regrowth of Kymi. This small town of ancient origins was all but lost during the wars which beset its mother country. For almost four hundred years, Kymi had suffered cultural and economic ruin at the hand of its Turkish overloads. Through the decades of unbridled power, these masters not only drained their fiefdoms of their wealth, but they had attempted to destroy all vestiges of Hellenism. As complacency and pleasure-seeking began to weaken many of these despots, Greek nationalism revived, culminating in the war for Greek liberation in 1821. The Greek forces in the lower peninsula, however, were more successful than their compatriots to the north, including those on the island of Euboea. This island, the largest in the Greek Archipelago, was located just off the Boeotian coast of Greece. Here attempts of the Greeks to expel the alien forces had been met with severe defeat. Shortly after the beginning of hostilities, Kymi was razed by the Turkish ruler of the district of Karistia, Omer Bey. As a result of this continued Turkish domination, Euboea was not included in the Greek territory liberated by the treaty of 1829. It was not until 1833 that annexation of the new Greek state was granted by Turkey in exchange for the island of Samos. The rebuilding of Kymi began

Supported in part by a grant from The American Cancer Society, Inc.

3

immediately after 1833 and the little town grew steadily through migration from within the island, as well as from the mainland of Greece. It was ideally situated, occupying the gently sloping hillsides of the Oxylithos and Kastrian Heights, which embrace a beautiful natural harbor as they slip beneath the sea. The town was rebuilt in amphitheater fashion overlooking the deep blue waters of the intruding Aegean Sea. Olive and fig trees and vineyards were planted in abundance. When the phylloxera had reduced the vineyards of France and Italy to only hope of survival, the vineyards of Kymi still flourished. At this time, her famous "black" wines, so called because of their intensely red color, were exported to ports around the world. In addition, coal, olive oil and figs became prime export items and gave to Kymi a modest maritime affluence at the end of the nineteenth century.

Kymi was generally a quiet town where life was casual and centered around the town square. Behind acacia trees lining the square were coffee shops, candy stores and produce markets. Political discussions, card games and Tavli (backgammon) were always to be found in the shops or around tables set among the trees. Thick black coffee or oozo were favorite beverages. Young people walked arm-in-arm through the city on cool evenings and the bozookia could be heard in the square or along the narrow streets. Fish and lobsters were abundant and each Saturday a public market was held with farmers from local villages bringing their produce to sell. A great Basilica, St. Athanasios, completed in 1869, dominated the eastern side of the square. Its seaward ramparts were bordered by multicolored flower gardens which were the site of community celebrations, especially on religious holidays. In August, the mass commemorating the Assumption of the Blessed Virgin and the ensuing gigantic banquet marked the most popular of Kymi's feastdays.

Many tourists visted Kymi to vacation along the coast where swimming, boating and seafood were available in a quaint and picturesque setting. Others made pilgrimages to Choneutikon, a well-known "healing spring" located below the town. Its medical qualities attracted many who, in search of health, would spend days or weeks living in the cottages and eating in the restaurant located near the spring.

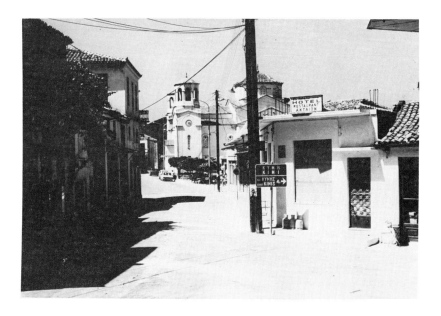

Figure 2. Entrance to the town of Kymi, Euboea, Greece, birthplace of Dr. Papanicolaou.

Nicholas Papanicolaou, son of Athanase, received the best education Greece could offer and, in addition, a modest material inheritance. A talented and ambitious student, he studied literature and philosophy, prior to receiving his medical education in Athens. Returning to the then thriving town of Kymi, he married Maria Kritsoutas in 1879.

Maria had been living with an aunt in Kymi following the death of her parents in Nauplia. Nauplia, the first post-revolutionary capital of Greece, had become the new nation's cultural and social center. Maria's father had been stationed as a military officer there. In Nauplia, she was exposed to great music and the classical literature of Greece, for which she retained an abiding love.

On May 13, 1883, a third child was born to Maria and Nicholas Papanicolaou. He was christened George Nicholas, being named for his father and maternal grandfather. All four children, Athanase, Maria, George and, finally, Helen, were born in the first family home located just below the courtyard of the Basilica of St. Athanasios. Shortly after the birth of Helen in 1886, Dr. Nicholas built a new three-story, stone-framed home facing directly east toward the harbor. It was in this close family unit, surrounded by the hills and seacoast of this town of about 8,000 inhabitants, that George Papanicolaou spent his early childhood.

When he reached the age of four and one-half years, young George entered the local grammar school. After-school hours were spent hiking in the nearby mountains or, more often, walking along the sea or boating. The young lad was quite sensitive and sentimental, frequently displaying a sad countenance and often crying. His father would jokingly say, "George, your face resembles a map," as the many tears made irregular lines across his face. Despite his rather fragile personality as a child, he was intent on superior physical development and the acquisition of courage. Considering boating both a pleasure and a challenge, he would often row out into the treacherous sea and wrestle with the waves to strengthen his endurance and bolster his courage. One stormy day he almost capsized, to the consternation of several towns-people who happened to witness the event from shore. So treacherous is the water along the coast of Kymi during certain seasons, that ship captains assiduously avoided the so-called

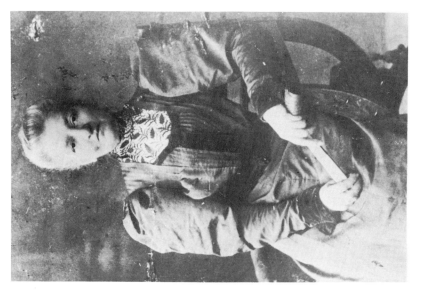

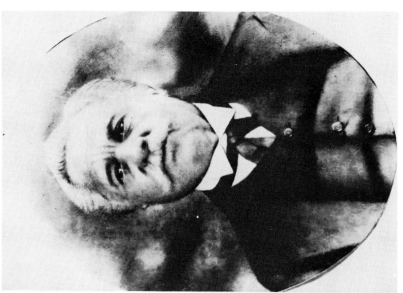

Figure 3. Nicholas and Mary Papanicolaou, parents of George N. Papanicolaou.

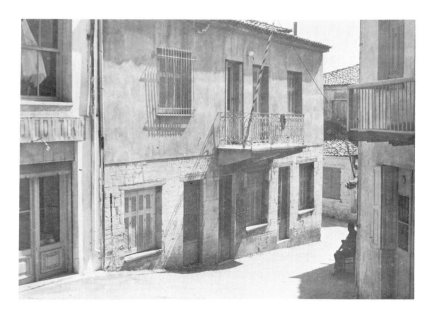

Figure 4. Birthplace and first home of George N. Papanicolaou, Kymi, Greece.

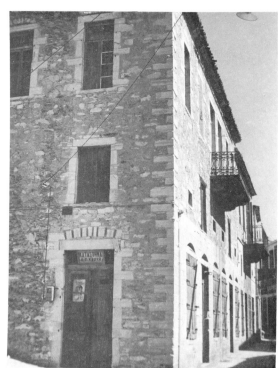

Figure 5. The second home of George Papanicolaou in Kymi, built by his father about 1886.

Kafireas. George had been warned but ignored the advice.

When he was not walking barefoot along the water's edge or boating, George would generally be found exploring the hills around the town. He loved nature and was curious concerning the plants and animals abounding in the surrounding hillsides. He and his friend would often become so absorbed in their exploration that they would walk for two or three hours without speaking to one another. Another of his pleasures was the enjoyment of a good book, usually a classical novel, while sitting secluded under a tree listening to the delightful sounds of nature.

The young lad was greatly influenced by his mother. In contrast to a rather stern and domineering father, his mother was mild and gentle. Her great love for music, literature and religion was conveyed to her children, broadening their cultural horizons and engendering personal ambition. This is not to imply that Maria Papanicolaou was not an active and energetic woman. She participated in community affairs and encouraged her children to follow her example. George sang in the church choir on special occasions and joined his mother in campaigning for Dr. Nicholas, who was elected Mayor of Kymi and on two occasions Senator to the Greek Congress from the district of Karistia. The young boy helped his father, as Mayor, lay the cornerstone at the dedication of the new harbor.

The Papanicolaou family enjoyed picnics. Their favorite picnic ground lay high on a northern cape which fell precipitously to the sea. It could be reached only by walking or traveling on donkey. On the path about half way to their destination, the seventeenth century Sacred Monastery of the Savior, white against the blue sky, lay isolated on the treeless mountainside. In this peaceful setting where silence was broken only by the bleating of a goat or the excited murmurings of a chicken, a demitasse of thick coffee was offered the weary traveler and the donkey was given rest and water. When finally the top of the cape was reached, one felt enraptured, sensing the lofty calmness as he looked for miles across the broad expanse of the Aegean. This spot would soon be missed, though it would play a significant role in the later life of the young boy.

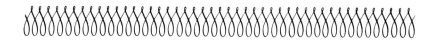

CHAPTER II

TO ATHENS FOR GYMNASIUM,
UNIVERSITY AND MEDICAL SCHOOL

REACHING age eleven years, he completed grammar school and had to prepare for the gymnasium. Kymi could not provide this higher education and the Papanicolaou children were sent to Athens. Though George wept as he said goodbye to his family and home, he was fortunate in being able to share a room with his older brother already in school in the ancient city. Until that time, Kymi had been George's only known world. But he soon· became acquainted with the large city and enjoyed the varied opportunities it offered, including violin lessons at the Lotner Conservatory of Music.

Nevertheless, he could not give up his longing for the sea, and at age thirteen years he attempted to join the navy. His efforts were thwarted since he was too young to take the examination. He soon forgot the navy as his intellectual interests broadened, especially after his family moved to Athens following the election of his father as Senator. His father was deeply interested in having his children appreciate their cultural heritage. He often strolled with them among the monuments of classical Greece, supplying the historical background and discussing the influence of that Golden Age on modern society. This he knew well for he loved his country.

Knowing his father's friendship with Premier Tricoupis, George asked to be allowed to speak to the Premier some day. Accordingly, his father arranged a meeting and, among other things, the Premier asked the young boy, "What are you going to be when you become a man?" Seeing his idol, the young student became timid. "I don't know yet," he replied, lost for words. "When I was your age, I knew this very well," replied Tricoupis

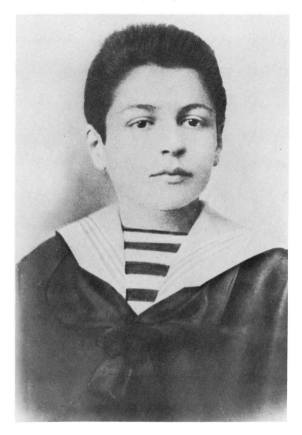

Figure 6. George N. Papanicolaou, age 13 years – the year he attempted to join the Greek navy.

with a smile. This encounter deeply impressed the youngster and awakened a sense of ambition which was to drive him the remainder of his life.

Since his older brother decided against medicine, Dr. Nicholas hoped that George would study medicine and return to Kymi to practice with him. The vistas, however, were too broad at this time to enable the student to decide what direction his life should take. He was greatly influenced by his association with Stephen Konstantinides, a relative with whom he lived for one year. Stephen had studied law in Germany and was a disciple of German culture.

In 1898 George Papanicolaou entered the University of Athens. Here he was given the freedom to pursue his innate interests, the humanities and music. Being an avid reader, he became acquainted with the new philosophical thinking current at the close of the nineteenth century. Soon he mastered French, then still the international language, and he continued his study of the violin, which became an enduring source of pleasure. His various cultural pursuits were expensive. George's father, having to support four children, complained of his son's heavy expenditures, but George felt that anything which contributed to his culture was indispensable.

Beside being intellectually stimulating, university life for the affluent student could also be carefree. However, money sometimes did become scarce. On these occasions, George and his friends would dine with simple food and cheap wine in an atmosphere of elegance created by his background music. Frequent parties also lent a certain gaiety to life and George Papanicolaou was very much a part of these activities.

But he soon became concerned about the future. Though he was never enthusiastic about becoming a practicing physician, he was encouraged to study medicine by his father. Thus, apparently more from loyalty to his father rather than personal desire, George Papanicolaou entered medical school. He pursued his scientific studies in earnest and in 1904 at age twenty-one years, he graduated grade "A."

Following the completion of his medical studies, George was called to military service on October 3, 1904, in the 3rd regiment of infantry. On October 14, 1904, he was admitted to the school for reserve officers and approximately two weeks later, he was named "auxiliary nurse." In January 1906, the young officer was promoted to assistant surgeon and remained in this capacity until completion of his military obligation on August 15, 1906. At this time, his father tried to persuade his son to remain in the army as a physician, but the young man became angry, stating he was looking forward to a career of scientific research.

During his early months in the army, George Papanicolaou wrote the following letter to his father. [The young physician had asked his father for financial support to allow him to continue his

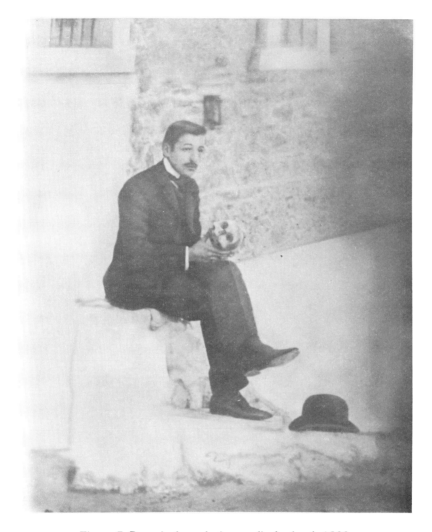

Figure 7. Papanicolaou during medical school, 1903.

education outside Greece. He was not interested in returning to Kymi to establish a private practice. His father, who had spent considerable time away from his profession in order to engage in politics, felt that he must consider the needs of his children equally. Too, he considered further education for the young physician as impractical. In reply to his son, Dr. Nicholas

Papanicolaou suggested that George become a military physician. This reply incensed his ambitious and now self-confident son and set the stage for a breach between them which was never fully healed.]

December 31, 1904

My respected father:

Day before yesterday, I received your letter and the fifty drachmas. I was very saddened though with all that you wrote me. Not only was I saddened but frightened. With this blow that I received, I can truthfully say that I felt deeply the true meaning of fear. Something that at any other period in my life I could ignore, today I feel my knees buckling under me. I must stand by and watch all my dreams be destroyed one by one. I must bow to the fate that means my disaster, my ruin. That is what your letter said to me. A spirit of disappointment, disillusionment and despair covers all of your words. I must be subjected to your will. For the first time in my life reality stands naked before my eyes.

The voice inside of me then was false – for it kept telling me, "Go forward." It was false because it has been saying, "For the brave traveler, there are no limits, no set boundaries," but now I hear another harsh voice saying to me, "Unlimited is a word for the free. You were born bound tightly with obligation. Do you see that wall? That is the grave of your impossible dreams."

I don't want to be a military doctor. No! I don't want that! I want to be free. I want to feel all the joy that the battle of life has to offer. Only the weak and the cowardly seek the harbors. But for me, there is no fear of the open sea. I want my freedom, that sweet freedom that I need to fight whatever tries to crush me. The trumpet of battle is like a sweet lullaby to my soul, because in battle all of the decayed ghosts die to make room for the healthy new life that appears. I dream of this battle because the battle is also the joy of life. I want my weapons now. I need them for the combat that beckons me. That is what I'm asking of you. Come now! Why do you look at me like this? Do you not have what I'm asking for? And if not, what of it? I shall never enter the harbor – never! Do you understand me? Never! I am not a coward. It is better for me to be destroyed, erased, than to have my soul say, "Wait! Enough of dreaming. Obligation is speaking, not your wishes." Shall I stop? No, for my will shall never speak to me like this. Like a stone wall it will confront this obligation and it will conquer – yes, it will conquer.

In your youth you were wealthy, educated, well-bred. You were the image of an era. You reached a respectable height. You served society according to your conception of life of that time. You lived that way and you continue to live that way until this day. And if you refuse to weaken today, this is due to your unchanging nature, as well as to your resistance to the natural law for change and for anything new.

I am your son – and as your son, I must follow you faithfully. I must be active today as you were active – though a different road for the same goal. This is the most crucial period of my life. Today I am on trial. Don't mention to me again what you have said up to now, because should I live my life as you wish, I am completely destroyed.

Don't try to take away the strength that I have left, but try to strengthen me with your strength. What good would one hundred or five hundred or one thousand drachmas be to me (if I could raise that much). No! Even you would not like that. If I were completely exhausted financially maybe I would speak differently to you. Now, though, I think it is a sin to be sacrificed.

Help me. Try to give something so that we may get out of this hopeless situation. Don't procrastinate. Let all of your thoughts revolve around that. I don't care if I suffer one or two or three months. It is all right. I'll gladly suffer so long as I don't lose hope that I'll be able to follow the road that I have mapped out with so much longing. I know my future. I only ask for the means from you. Come! Do not forsake me. Have compassion for me. Help me all you can. Use whatever means remain and rest assured you will never regret whatever you do.

> With unlimited respect,
> Your Son, George

Returning home after serving his military obligation, Papanicolaou was expected to join his father in the practice of medicine; however, his mind was concerned with other matters. He had always been disturbed that his father with such broad educational and intellectual interests had returned to his small, somewhat isolated hometown to practice medicine. Settled in Kymi, he would find himself out of the mainstream of knowledge. There would be few people with whom to discuss the fascinating philosophical and scientific developments of the day. Beside the fear of cultural isolation, the young physician had little interest in the practice of medicine. His father was concerned and wondered what would become of this young man with such an "unsettled" mind. He would see his son walking along the beach, studying philosophical dissertations without any apparent practical goal, or find that he was up on the hillside under the trees reading Goethe or Nietzsche. George made no attempt to establish an office and refused to engage in medical practice on a routine basis. Even the townsfolk were disturbed that a young man with a medical education would not desire to practice medicine. For this reason, he was considered by many townspeople to be odd, though no one doubted his exceptional ability.

Among the few attended professionally by the new Dr. Papanicolaou were the poor lepers whose colony was located along the coast twenty miles north of Kymi near the well-known rock formation called Kalogiros, or the Priest. Except for food and other goods left for them by generous townsfolk, these neglected people had little other contact with the community. Although a physician was supposed to attend their needs, they received little care. The sympathetic Papanicolaou visited them frequently and it was not uncommon for persons living near the road to the colony to hear one of the diseased individuals calling for the new physician to come help. He always responded.

During this year of indecision and intellectual searching, a very fortunate acquaintance was made. A branch of the famous military family, Mavroyeni, moved from Athens to Kymi to spend summer vacation each year. During the summer of 1906, a young daughter in the family became ill. A neighbor was asked to recommend a local physician and she advised that the new Dr. Papanicolaou be called. The Papanicolaou family had known the Mavroyenis since calling on them shortly after the newcomers bought their first home near the coast. After the professional consultation, Dr. Papanicolaou refused to charge a fee because, as he stated, the families were close friends. It was at this time that he first met Mary Mavroyeni. She was already a close friend of his sister, Helen. From that time, Mary was always included in the Papanicolaou family excursions and picnics.

Becoming more and more absorbed with philosophy and new theories concerning the biological sciences, George Papanicolaou asked his father to allow him to go to Germany for further study. Realizing that he was a sentimental person, Papanicolaou was afraid that this trait would handicap his decisions and career. He struggled to overcome his sentimentality, believing that an ambitious man must fight to achieve his goals. Philosophy, he felt, could help him overcome this weakness. He had become intrigued with the writings of Goethe, Nietzsche, Kant, Schopenhauer and Haeckel. Ernst Haeckel's *Riddle of the Universe,* published in 1898, had captured a large audience throughout the world. It dealt with the immensely popular subject of Darwin's theory of evolution and Haeckel had added his own monistic concept in an effort to bring unity to philosophy and the biological sciences. Haeckel occupied the Chair of Anthropology at the University of Jena. Finally realizing that his talented son could not be swayed and that he indeed had no interest in medical practice, Dr. Nicholas conceded and George was soon accepted for postgraduate study in Jena, Germany.

Before leaving Greece, there was one thing which George Papanicolaou was determined to do. This concerned an operation to have his slight bowleg condition corrected. He consulted Professor Chrysospathis, the leading orthopedic surgeon in Greece. The professor refused to consider surgery for so minimal an abnormality. Finally, George located a physician who would undertake the task. This was reported to his professor. Knowing the incompetency of the second physician, the professor agreed to perform the procedure himself. An osteotomy was usually performed and the patient was placed in bilateral leg casts for a short time thereafter. Information concerning the exact operation performed on Papanicolaou is not available. During the period of convalescence, the house next to the clinic was destroyed by fire and everyone left the clinic except for Papanicolaou, who was immobilized by leg casts. The clinic, however, escaped the fire and tragedy was averted. The operation was a success and pleased him immensely.

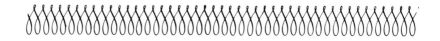

CHAPTER III

POSTGRADUATE STUDY IN GERMANY

THE nineteenth century was an exciting era in zoology. Probably nowhere was this science developing more rapidly than in Germany. In 1827 Von Baer discovered the mammalian ovum. Twelve years later, applying the discovery Schleiden made in botany, Theodor Schwann demonstrated the cell as the basic biological structure of the animal world. Virchow published a treatise on cellular pathology in 1858 and during the following decade, he applied the cellular theory to the human in all details, both in health and disease. He stated that all cells of all organisms arose from a single cell, the fertilized ovum. But it was not until 1875 that fertilization of an ovum was first observed by Oscar Hertwig, probably in collaboration with his brother, Richard.

August Weismann, through brilliant speculation, had concluded that all inheritance was transmitted by the sex cells only. The hereditary mechanism, he postulated, involved a series of molecular units placed along the chromosomes. His rejection of the inheritance of acquired characteristics added further controversy to a world already thrown into debate since Darwin's theory of evolution was expounded in 1859. This debate, for the most part, pitted science against the prevailing dogmas of Christianity. Ernst Haeckel tried to reconcile the problem through the formation of his monistic philosophy which he felt unified all knowledge. Rejecting immortality, he equated God and nature by stipulating that God exists only as the spiritual force which pervades all nature. At age twenty-nine years, as Extraordinaire Professor at the University of Jena, Haeckel had attacked the beliefs of his elders by drawing conclusions from the theory of evolution which Darwin himself hesitated to suggest. The young academician was the first to compile a genealogical tree of the relationships between the orders of animals. He emphasized the biogenetic law that ontogeny recapitulates phylogeny. In 1899 Haeckel defended his monistic concept at length in the immensely popular book, *Riddle of the Universe.* It was this book more than any other which persuaded George Papanicolaou to pursue a study of the philosophy of the biological sciences. Professor Haeckel had reached his seventy-third birthday by this time, but he still occupied the Chair of Zoology at Jena. Since it was customary for a student to choose his university according to the reputation of his desired professor, George requested and secured a post-graduate position under Ernst Haeckel.

In the spring of 1907, George Papanicolaou set out for Jena, Germany. The little town was a typical university community, mingling the "new and the old as none but the Germans know how to do."* With its casual cobblestone streets, Gothic churches and the river Salle drifting from among the Thurigian hills, it retained its medieval aspect. Papanicolaou must have thought of Goethe as he wandered through the streets among the oxen and horse-drawn carts and bicycles, for Goethe had composed the "Erlkönig" in Jena and the town had preserved his memory in Goethe Strasse. The students seemed aware of the university's 350 years of tradition as they swaggered through town in their bright-colored caps. As George attended the lectures, he must have ·oeen impressed with the vigor and self-assurance of his large-framed mentor who had endured the storm of controversy for the past forty-five years. However, the mental stimulation which he had hoped for was not there, and after one semester, he decided to move to Freiburg under the tutelage of August Weismann.

Weismann's theory of the continuity of germ plasm and the noninheritance of acquired characteristics had become the cornerstone of the modern science of genetics. He was the same age as Hackel, and defective vision hampered his work seriously. Although he found his work, even there, disappointing, it was during this period that George Papanicolaou determined to devote his life to biological research.

---

*Slosson: *Major Prophets of Today.* 1914, p. 245.

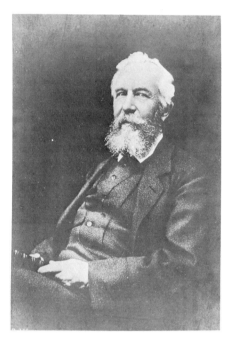

Figure 8. Prof. Ernst Haeckel of Jena, one of Europe's greatest early proponents of Darwinism and Papanicolaou's first teacher in Germany.

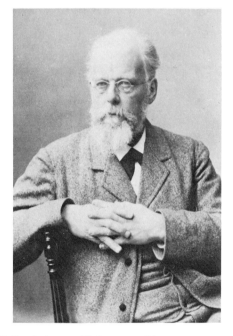

Figure 9. Prof. August Weismann of Freiburg, brilliant early geneticist.

Knowing of the great reputation enjoyed by Richard Hertwig, he decided to join him at the Zoological Institute in Munich after one semester in Freiburg. Papanicolaou was accepted as "Doktorand Nominally" of Richard Hertwig and was to begin work on generations of daphnia under the special supervision of Richard Goldschmidt.

Arriving in Munich, he procured a room at a boarding house. Students generally selected a room by wandering through town looking for notices on the homes. The availability of rooms for rent, as well as frequently the name of the occupant, were noted along the gutters of the houses. This allowed the foreign students on occasion to find a landlord of the same national heritage. Characteristically, the landlords charged the students rather heavy rental, especially if such comforts as indoor bathing facilities were furnished.

The Zoological Institute in Munich was considered to be the greatest zoological research center in the world at that time. It occupied a portion of the second floor of the old Academy, an eighteenth century monastery constructed in quadrangular fashion with a series of courtyards. The student laboratory consisted of a single large room with a vaulted ceiling, supported by marble columns. Three large windows provided a beautiful view of the nave of St. Michael's Church, behind which could be seen the two famous onion towers of Our Lady's Cathedral. As had been customary for decades, priests from nearby St. Michael's Church could still be seen walking about, taking care of their rose gardens. Beside the large research laboratory, there were three offices and the two rooms of Professor Hertwig, which together comprised the Institute's quarters. Along this row of rooms stretched a long corridor with numerous windows looking toward another courtyard.

Though the fixtures and apparatus were very poor, a wonderful spirit prevailed and the kind professor inspired his students with a love for research. The student was given his problem, laboratory supplies and reading material and then allowed to work as quickly or slowly as he cared. The professor and instructors made daily rounds, answered questions, discussed technique and suggested pertinent references in the literature. As the student mastered one

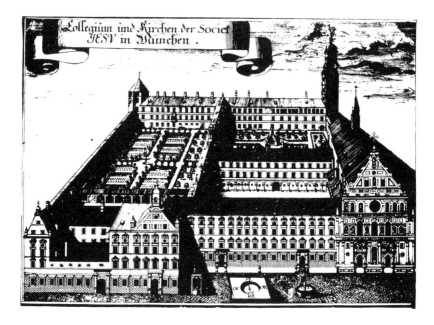

Figure 10. The old Academy Munich: formerly a monastery, it later housed
the Hertwig Zoological Institute.

topic, he was presented with another until the whole field of
zoology had been covered. Generally, a student had to look
forward to two years of detailed study before receiving his Ph.D.
Time requirements were flexible, however, allowing a student to
proceed at his own speed.

Dr. Goldschmidt, in addition to his routine consultations, held
a daily tea table for student discussion. Once weekly, all students
and associates of Dr. Hertwig gathered for a seminar. Each student
had to report on the progress with his delegated work while others
in attendance were encouraged to participate in discussion.

Attendance at lectures was required and it was necessary to
spend considerable time in the laboratory where the teaching staff
could review the student's work often. This frequent reappraisal of
progress eventually served to enhance the acceptance of the
student's thesis. Due to the large number of international visitors,
in addition to the doctoral candidates, twenty or thirty students
might be crowded into the Institute.

Papanicolaou was assigned a problem involving sex differentiation and sex determination of daphina, a subject suggested by Dr. Hertwig. Dr. Hertwig conceived the idea that sex determination might be related to the nucleoplasmic ratio of the gametes. This speculation led to large-scale experiments by Hertwig and his students, including Papanicolaou, on sex determination in a variety of organisms. As was soon learned, however, sex determination was not related to the nucleoplasmic ratio but could be understood only genetically. Although this earlier concept was found to be invalid, Hertwig received lasting acclaim for his development of the germ layer theory and his priority in demonstrating the artificial induction of parthenogenesis in the sea urchin egg.

As indicative of the research atmosphere to which Papanicolaou was exposed during his study in Munich might be cited the traditional event known as "fertilization day." Dr. Goldschmidt describes the preparation as a period of great exitement, awaiting the arrival of the crates of sea urchins which had to be shipped in local sea water from the Mediterranean. Immediately after unpacking, fertilization tests were made and then periodically thereafter until the appropriate day arrived. On that day. Dr. Hertwig reported to the laboratory at 7:00 A.M., made final preparations, and at 2:00 P. M. personally placed sea urchin eggs under the microscope of each student so that the fertilization process could be observed. This laboratory demonstration not only vividly illustrated a fascinating biological process, but mimicked the experiment by which his brother, Oscar Hertwig, had established that fertilization is essentially the fusion of two nuclei – that of the egg and that of the sperm.

Dr. von Frisch, a fellow student with Papanicolaou and later successor to Dr. Hertwig, describes Papanicolaou as a kind person, exhibiting fast, adroit movements and one always ready for discussion at the daily tea table of Richard Goldschmidt. Papanicolaou bred daphnia in drinking glasses placed in large gas-heated tin troughs of water. It was common to see him, waiter-like, balancing trays with fifty or more glasses as he passed through the corridor on his way back to the laboratory. His research required that he isolate each parthenogenic daughter of

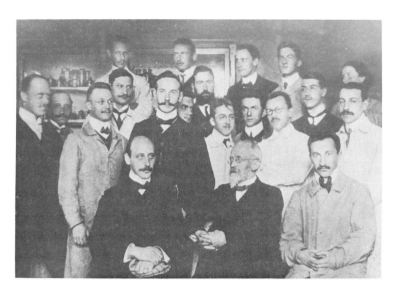

Figure 11. Front row, l to r, Dr. Richard Goldschmidt, Dr. R. Hertwig, Dr. M. Popoff. Papanicolaou stands, second row, far right, and Dr. Karl von Frisch is standing last row, far left. Hertwig Institute, 1909.

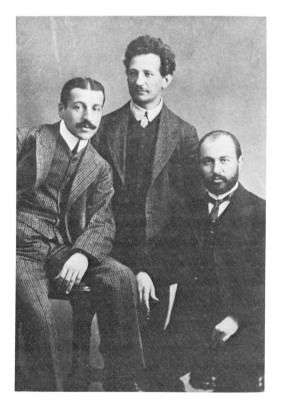

Figure 12. Papanicolaou with Greek friends in Germany around 1910.

his one female in a special glass.

At the daily tea table, plans for the following weekend were usually made. Munich had much to offer a student. Heated discussions of art and literature enlivened the coffee houses; new types of poetry and the graphic arts were being fostered. Concerts, where students were given preference in the standing area, could be enjoyed and the Alps invited skiing in the winter and hiking in the summer. This was the type of life which Papanicolaou relished. He was somewhat older and more mature than many of the other students, for he had studied medicine, served in the army and consumed part of a year reading at home before coming to Germany. Prof. O. Koehler of Freiburg describes him as knowing "a lot of medicine and international politics and being a good comrade at the tea table and skiing."

During the Easter vacation of 1909, Papanicolaou and Karl von Frisch took the marine training course available at the Zoological Station at Trieste. This was a state-supported research station directed by the Austro-Hungarian monarchy. It was common for zoological students studying in the inland areas to spend time along the waterfront to observe marine specimens. At Trieste, daily lectures were given by Professor Corey, described as a most knowledgeable and stimulating teacher. He also captained the boat which took the students on marine excursions along the beautiful Dietrian and Dalmatian coasts which abounded in aquatic life.

Papanicolaou contracted malaria during his stay in Germany. Whether or not it occurred during this trip to Trieste is unknown, but malaria was endemic on the western Adriatic coast of Austria.

Trips such as the one to Trieste were probably financed by Papanicolaou himself. Since graduate students were expected to be self-supporting, they were dependent on family resources or outside income. Dr. Papanicolaou was provided with sufficient funds to enjoy recreational activities, as well as to pursue his education. He accumulated a large wardrobe of fine suits to insure a proper appearance for social functions. He was able to enjoy to the fullest the excitement of living in Munich, described by Richard Goldschmidt as representing "the artistic center of Germany, combining the charming levity of Vienna, the Bohemian extravagance of Paris, the happy-go-lucky life of Florence and

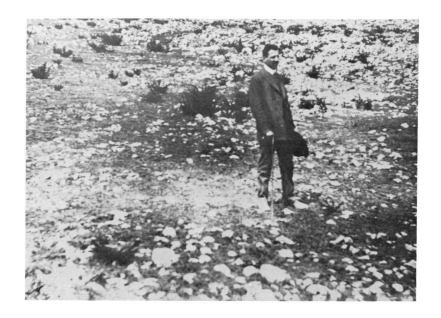

Figure 13. George Papanicolaou in the Karst Mountains near Trieste, April, 1909. Photo courtesy of Dr. Karl von Frisch.

Naples, all with its beautiful location in the grand Isar Valley near the Alps."

By 1910, Papanicolaou had completed his study and was prepared to present his thesis. The Ph.D. candidate was required to visit each of the four professors who would examine him and present each a copy of his thesis and an invitation to his lecture. This traditional task had to be performed in full regalia, including top hat. At 10:00 A.M. on the designated day, the candidate, again dressed in formal evening attire, presented his thesis in the large lecture hall. The room was usually empty except for a few friends and students and the examining professors. The doctoral candidate, after his presentation, might be required to elaborate more fully or defend certain points. The professors then briefly discussed his performance and rendered their verdict.

After obtaining his Ph.D., Dr. Papanicolaou departed for Greece, hoping to embark on an academic career there.

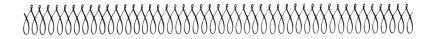

CHAPTER IV

OCEANOGRAPHIC MUSEUM-MONACO

 M UCH to Papanicolaou's disappointment, he "found conditions in Greece unfavorable to a continuation of biological research which had now become my chief concern." At that time there was only one university (Athens) and laboratory facilities were scarce and inadequate in his native country. Papanicolaou was offered a position in the university, which he declined because of the poor potential for an academic career. It must be remembered that at this time Hellenism was in a state of crisis. Half of the Greek people were still under Ottoman domination and the "young Turk" movement which began in 1908 had attempted to further destroy Greek national life. The country was poor and the government unstable. Notable, however, was the fact that Venizelos, a potential patron and Greek nationalist, took office as Premier during the fall of 1910. But Papanicolaou had already departed. The young scientist had concluded that he must leave Greece to seek an academic career.

First he visited Kymi. Dr. Nicholas had selected the daughter of a wealthy merchant in Kymi for George to marry. Some minor dispute apparently had arisen concerning the dowry but this was soon settled. George Papanicolaou, however, found the whole affair unpleasant and decided to leave Greece immediately. He unexpectedly traveled in the company of the Mavroyeni family, including Mary, on the ferry from Eritrea to the Greek mainland. Mary was playing the piano and Papanicolaou, who had his violin with him, accompanied her. The Mavroyenis were returning to Athens following their annual summer vacation in Kymi.

This fortunate encounter with Mary set the stage for one of the most important events in the life of the scientist. Visiting in the Mavroyeni home on several occasions during his wait to return to

Europe, he became quite fond of Mary. Rapidly becoming more serious in his affection for her, he wanted them to be alone, but this was impossible in her home because of the social custom of that time. Finally, George persuaded her to meet him along the street near a relative's home. On the second such meeting he asked her to marry him. Mary agreed. Col. Mavroyeni's consent was obtained and immediate plans for the wedding were made. Mary Mavroyeni and George Papanicolaou were married in a small private ceremony by an Orthodox priest at the bride's home on September 25, 1910. Dr. Papanicolaou's parents and relatives were unaware of the marriage at that time, as George knew that his father would disapprove vigorously.

Since dowries for daughters of military men were provided by the government, Mary's dowry was very small. The total allotment by the government for all dowries during the year was predetermined, so that the amount of each individual dowry was based on the number of weddings taking place during that year. Col. Mavroyeni provided first-class passage for the couple, who sailed on the liner, Athenai, for Marseilles with little more than Mary's small dowry to sustain them during their combined honeymoon and search for employment.

From Marseilles they boarded a train which took them along the Cote d'Azur, stopping at Cap T'antibe and Nice. In Nice the parade of flowers was in progress with young girls dressed in colorful gay costumes. After a brief visit there, the couple proceeded by streetcar to the marine laboratory in Ville Franche. This Russian biological station was housed in an old prison which lent a somber atmosphere with its vestiges of a not-too-pleasant past. Fishermen would bring marine specimens each morning. The area was especially rich in plankton but large snails, ten to fifteen inches in length, and transparent vividly colored jelly fish might be seen. The Papanicolaous stayed in the best hotel in town for the equivalent of about "seventy-five cents" daily, which included room, board and unlimited wine. An active night life in the little village was insured by the presence of sailors who were given shore leave while their ships were in harbor.

Leaving Ville Franche, the couple continued by tram to Monaco. The Oceanographic Museum there had been dedicated in

February. It received wide acclaim as one of the finest marine research stations in the world. Prince Albert I of Monaco had long been interested in oceanographic research. Beginning about 1885, he had made periodic excursions on his various yachts to collect marine specimens for analysis and classification. The 1901 expedition was notable in that Drs. Portier and Richet made a study of the toxic properties of the jelly fish Physalias. During these experiments, performed on board the yacht, the two scientists proved that an aqueous glycerin extract of the filaments of Physalia was extremely toxic to ducks and rabbits. On returning to France they had difficulty in obtaining Physalia but continued their experiments, using extracts from Actinaria which resembled Physalia and were more easily procured. While studying the effects of this toxin on dogs, Portier and Richet discovered the anaphylactic phenomenon which they described and named in 1902.

Such scientific naval expeditions were not unusual. One recalls Charles Darwin's five-year voyage on the "Beagle," (1830-1836) which took him to many lands and acquainted him with ancient biological forms. From these investigations he later derived his theory of evolution. The British ship, "Challenger," had pulled many intriguing inhabitants from the deep sea in the period 1872-1876, and just prior to the Papanicolaous' visit, Charcot (son of the famous J. M. Charcot of Paris) had returned from the antartic with penguins for the museum in Monaco. For a biologist on tour, Monaco was a must.

The museum was built along the edge of a large rock formation which fell abruptly to the Mediterranean. The halls in the museum were adorned with penguins, the bony remains of whales and various other forms of aquatic life. In the large colonnaded entrance hall was a gigantic chandelier in the form of a jelly fish, reminiscent of the work of Portier and Richet.

Marine research involving live specimens was carried out in the many laboratories containing huge aquariums. While walking through one of the corridors, Papanicolaou met an old friend from Germany who was employed by the museum as a physiologist. He was leaving December thirty-first and suggested that Papanicolaou apply for his job. The proposition was considered. Papanicolaou was not especially interested in marine zoology, but he thought he might be able to accompany the Prince on his deep-sea expedition scheduled for the following summer. His German friend introduced him to Dr. Richard, director of the museum, and Papanicolaou's application for employment was accepted.

During his continuing travels, Papanicolaou wrote his parents on October 4, 1910, apparently confirming reports of his marriage to Mary. He emphasized that he would derive pleasure in life not primarily through achieving wealth or physical comfort, but by losing himself in some creative effort through which he could make a worthy contribution to life.

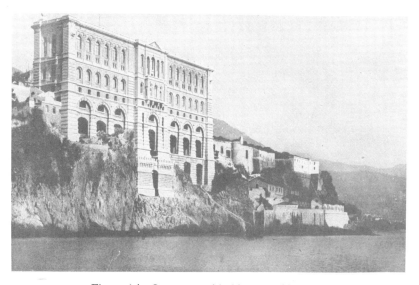

Figure 14. Oceanographic Museum, Monaco.

October 4, 1910

My respected parents:

I received your latest letters and was touched by the love you always continue to show me.

I feel though that I must confess that this excessive love for me makes me sad, because it is impossible for me to respond to it as I would like if I were independent. But now I find it necessary to add new sorrows to you — this time much larger — and I shall make you shed new tears. You should not hold this against me. You must know that anything I do does not emanate from egotism but from an inner need according to my personality – this need which urges to live, not to enjoy life, but to serve it. That which is enjoyment, for me it is hateful, and that is why I think it is my duty, collecting all of my strength, to choke all the feelings that interfere with my higher development. And I can follow freely the road that will lead me to the far removed point that I have set as a goal for my career.

It is not my ideal to be wealthy or to live happily, but to work to create – to do something worthy of a strong moral man. Is that my fault? Or is it something worthy of congratulations? Neither one nor the other. Both would be very subjective for me. All of them are necessary. I could not be anyone or anything else because I was born with these qualities. That is why I belive that I will succeed – in that case. I have hopes that some day I shall see you once more before we part forever, and with this hope I come now to bid you goodbye with tears in my eyes, hoping and praying that God will keep us in good health so that in the future we may be able to meet once more for the comfort and happiness of us all. Receive my warmest kisses and love, with sincere devotion and unlimited respect.

From your son,
George

Since he would not begin his work until January 1, 1911, the couple visited Paris in the interim. Almost continuous rains disturbed the travelers in Paris but they made good use of their time. Mary waited patiently during the many hours that George spent visiting the Louvre. The sidewalk cafes provided "atmosphere" and relief from the rigorous tourist routine.

Hoping also to see the famous butterfly collection of Prince Bonaparte while he was there, George visited the Prince's mansion and left his name with the secretary. Much to the excitement of the concierge of the small hotel where the Papanicolaous were staying, the Prince, in turn, called and left his card for Dr. Papanicolaou, who promptly visited him. Prince Roland Bonaparte was a patron of the natural sciences. His mansion contained one of the most beautiful private libraries anywhere. The reception room was a quadrangle of broad galleries, stacked to the ceiling with luxuriously bound books. The center of the room was occupied by antique tables on which were old globes and nautical instruments. George, himself a butterfly collector, always remembered that memorable day with his noble and hospitable host. It was somewhat later that Papanicolaou learned that Prince George of Crete, who married Prince Bonaparte's daughter and was living in Paris, was quite upset and embarrassed that his countryman would call on a foreign dignitary without paying respects to his own nobility.

Suddenly a severe bout of tonsilitis, an old enemy, struck Papanicolaou and caused the couple to return to Monaco after a rather brief stay in Paris. In Monaco the Papanicolaous located a comfortable apartment facing the sea. Excursions to nearby resort towns or hikes in the surrounding hills, plus an occasional visit to the casino, occupied them until the new year. As scheduled, Dr. Papanicolaou began work at the museum on January 1, 1911. He was hired as a "preparateur" and soon grew restless because his work became routine and monotonous and apparently was not concerned with a specific research effort. His employment was not time-consuming, however, and he was able to spend many happy hours with Mary, taking excursions to Mentone, Nice and Cannes, and the picturesque environs along the Riviera. Gambling at the casino was forbidden employees of the museum, but they were provided two free tickets each month to the concerts held in the large hall nearby. It was fortunate that the newlyweds had so much time together in which to enjoy each other, their associates at the museum and life along the Cote d'Azur. For once George Papanicolaou launched into his scientific research again, he would become totally committed to it, allowing himself only minimum time for rest and relaxation.

In the spring of 1911, Mary studied cooking at Monastier, France, near Lyon. During this period of loneliness Papanicolaou wrote to his sister, Nina.

March 8, 1911

My little Nina,

I am a little late in answering because of many worries and illnesses and so I believe you will forgive me. And then, too, the company of my dear Mary made me forget a number of my responsibilities. Now though that Mary has gone, and I am again alone – oh, that unbearable loneliness – now I begin out of necessity to be more orderly.

Your letter made me very happy, especially the few words from our dear Costee. He was right to be disappointed that I didn't invite him to my wedding, although he was in Athens. And then he knows it was not from lack of love and esteem, but only from fear that maybe he would proceed to telegraphic operations and cause unpleasant incidents, because you know, Nina, I have a very stubborn head. I think I'm wise – that I know it all – that I never make mistakes – and whatever I decide, it is the best and it must be done without fail. That is my biggest fault. Although at the same time, I think it is my greatest good trait, because without it I would not have the resoluteness and self-confidence that characterize me.

You see, everything in the world is divided, and the best traits walk hand in hand with the greatest faults. Anyhow, you know that I am sincere, harmless and with a heart not so hard as some of my actions seem to imply. I love and I grieve as the tenderest and the most sentimental man. That is why I suffer more and I cannot be happy even for a little while, because I have a restless mind, ambitious, harsh and always it wants something – always torturing me with its excessive requests.

Now I am married and one would think I married to live a more contented life, but look, I have managed to send Mary away and now I am alone and I suffer ten times more because I miss the companionship that eased and relieved me so much. And do you think that I will be satisfied with her schooling at Monastier? You will see that afterward I shall want to send her somewhere else – to Germany, to Switzerland, or I don't know where, to supplement her knowledge and her education.

And for what, you will ask me, when all of these things destroy my happiness and make me constantly miserable. And do I know? Even my heart wonders and asks, but my brain orders without condescending to give reasons for its high-handedness. Sometimes it is justified but the justifications are false, as are all justifications. You see, Nina, the human form is inexhaustible, peculiar, and each individual is an unsolved problem – mysterious. All of us move according to his character – slaves and instruments of one's needs and the strength that resides inside of us – and apparently only in this way is one free and self-existing.

That is how I act, not knowing why and not being able to act differently. Only after my every deed, I sit and think what excuse I can find to justify my actions.

If you were to carefully psychoanalyze yourself you will see that you don't do any better. That's why I don't find it logical to hold any hatred against anyone. It seems to me that everything in life is forgiven and anyone who has the strength and the power to forgive will never be found in a position to repent – ever.

I kiss all of you – you, Costa, Maria, Toula and Vaugelaki.

With much love,
Your George

Papanicolaou had hoped to be allowed to accompany Prince Albert on his oceanographic expedition scheduled for the summer of 1911. In fact, it was this possibility which had prompted him to apply for work at the museum. He repeatedly sought an answer from Dr. Richard, but each time was told that his request had not been approved. Suddenly on the morning of July 19, 1911, the day Prince Albert was to sail, Papanicolaou was notified by Dr. Richard that his request to join the research team had been accepted. He was advised to pack immediately. Mary telegraphed a friend in Geneva to obtain an apartment for her and she left for Switzerland.

A new steamship, replacing the Princess Alice II, had been constructed for the Prince at La Seyne Shipyard. The Prince christened his new vessel "The Hirondelle II." It was sleek, displaced 600 tons and was capable of a speed of 15 knots. Apart from the crew, those participating in the expedition were Prince Albert, Dr. Richard; Lt. Commander Bouree, an oceanographer; Gorin, an algologist; Tinayre, the artist; and Papanicolaou, physiologist. There was much work for all on board, for these voyages were planned and executed with care by the Prince. They were concerned with obtaining deep sea marine specimens, devising apparatus for deep sea research and introducing new methods of marine investigation. The principal goal of the 1911 cruise was "to explore intermediary depths of bathypelagic forms with a Bouree net."*

Departing Monaco on July 19, the expedition was concerned with exploration of sea life in the Mediterranean for the first week. A rather rigorous schedule was required for all of those on board. Following breakfast every morning, the Prince met with his

---

*S.A.S. Prince Albert I of Monaco: *Bulletin De L'Institut Oceonographique*, No. 234, June 12, 1912.

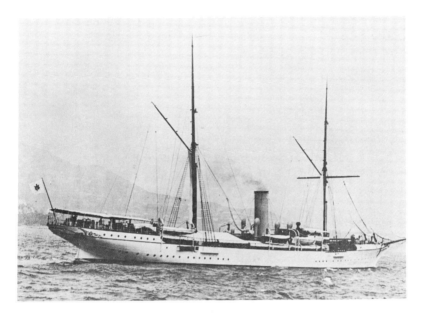

Figure 15. L'Hirondelle II, oceanographic vessel of Prince Albert I, Monaco, on which Papanicolaou acted as physiologist during the 1911 expedition.

collaborators at 8:00 A.M. and concluded plans for the research activities of the day.

The first maneuver consisted of sounding the depth of the sea. A net was then lowered and dragged as the ship moved slowly along. Marine specimens were obtained at various depths and then presented to Dr. Papanicolaou in the laboratory for examination and classification. Since unusual forms of sea life were encountered in a fresh state, work on board The Hirondelle II was more stimulating than that at the museum.

At lunch time everyone went downstairs and sat around the table with the Prince presiding. Although the Prince demanded unqualified respect, he permitted a certain casualness to encourage conversation. Several courses of delicious food were served at each luncheon. Usually the observations of the morning were discussed during this hour. The Prince was always served first, then each person in order of rank. By the time each course reached Papanicolaou, Prince Albert had already finished and the plates were being removed to make room for the next course. Due to this ritual, Papanicolaou occasionally missed portions of his meals and he attributed his striking weight loss during the expedition in part to this.

After the lunch hour everyone returned to work and on occasion pursued his research into the night. One night after the activities of the day had subsided, Papanicolaou decided to go on deck after 9:00 P.M. which, unknown to him, was against the protocol established by the Prince. On Papanicolaou's arrival the Prince turned to him but was silent and acted as if he did not notice him. Papanicolaou, uncertain concerning the meaning of this action, quietly left and returned below deck. A salon was provided there where one could read, play cards, relax and enjoy the company of others.

Two weeks were spent near Madeira and the Canary Islands, and then The Hirondelle II turned west to the Azores in search of whales. When one of the great cetaceans was located, the boat was lowered and the whaleman embarked with haste. The Prince took a position in the front of the ship behind the cannon which would fire the harpoon. After the animal was wounded with the first harpoon, it plunged, taking up the slack in the rope attached to the weapon. Soon though, it was obliged to resurface to breathe and a second harpoon killed it. Being brought on board, the animal was dissected by Papanicolaou. Undigested fragments of great cephalapods were often found in the stomachs of these large creatures. The swallowed specimens were of special interest since they could not otherwise be obtained.

At each of the ports Prince Albert sent telegrams to the families of his crew. In addition he paid all expenses while they were ashore including excursions in the environs of the ports. The Prince was respected not only because of his noble rank and dedication to oceanography, but also because of the kindness and thoughtfulness shown to those who worked with him. He was formal, however, in his relationships to the expedition's staff.

Returning to Monaco in September, The Hirondelle II anchored at Toulon to allow the Prince to proceed more directly to Paris. Dr. Papanicolaou who again had become ill with tonsillitis telegraphed Mary to meet him in Toulon. She immediately left

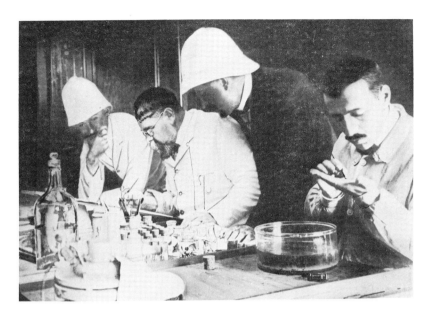

Figure 16. On board the L'Hirondelle II, 1911. Papanicolaou far right.

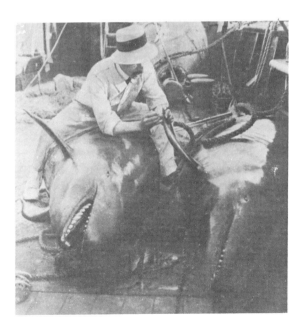

Figure 17. Papanicolaou labeling deep sea specimen, *Pseudorca crassidens,* the False Killer Whale. (Identification was made by Faith Turnbull of the International Oceanographic Foundation and later confirmed in *Bulletin De L'Institute Oceanographique* No. 234, June 12, 1912.

Geneva by train and arrived at 10:00 P.M. Being able to speak French with a local gendarme, she deposited her baggage in the train depot and set out with the policeman in a small boat for The Hirondelle II. She visited her feverish husband in his cabin and they decided to proceed to Monaco by train. Potassium chlorate appeared to relieve his sore throat and he soon became comfortable again. Mary was appalled at his weight loss of 20 pounds.

After returning to Monaco, Dr. Papanicolaou received a letter from his father requesting that they return to Kymi. Dr. Papanicolaou's mother had died during the earlier part of the year. His father was anxious to be with his children again. Dr. Papanicolaou completed his year assignment and the couple departed for Greece.

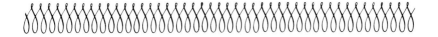

CHAPTER V

THE BALKAN WAR

AFTER a few months with his family in Greece, Papanicolaou left Mary in Kymi and returned to Germany and Monaco for about three months of additional study. The exact reason for this period of study is unknown, but the scientist seemed to have been amply gratified by this effort as expressed in another letter to Nina in June 1912.

June 22, 1912

My dear Nina,

On the first Saturday I wrote to Helen. This Saturday I'm writing to you, both times with the strains of music. At this moment I'm hearing the quadrille or cantata from "Carmen." Every now and then I feel a hard jarring that shows that an exceptional enthusiasm moves the emotions of the dancers and do you think the dancers are few? – about 300 young men and women. You can imagine the commotion! The entire hotel is in an uproar.

When I returned from Monaco at 7:30 P.M. the entertainment had not begun. I took a walk in the woods and saw the purple hues of the sun set back of the little village church. I then returned to drink my milk as I do every night. But when I returned to the hotel, I heard the beautiful sound of the violin and piano coming from the large auditorium and instead of going to my room I went directly to the hotel gardens where I ordered a glass of beer, some Vienese sausage and Chouchoute, and there I reminisced. I turned my thoughts back and looked at my life that had passed by as one agonizing effort. And for what? Why? Even I don't know. I had to become thirty years old to actually feel life and I had to return to Germany to see my life open like a flower in the sun.

But I find it is not too late. Doesn't the butterfly crawl for many months as a caterpillar before she wings? I feel as if I awakened from a deep sleep; that I am liberated from a tyrannical nightmare, so that I may follow the life that up until now I have looked on with contempt. It was these ideals that forced me to crawl like a caterpillar. I have thrown them away here in the waters of Isari and with them I have drowned the sorrow and the melancholia that have been my companions until now.

Idealism is the denial of life. Life is pulsation, vibration, sentiment and emotion. Meditations and endeavors are means, not goals or purposes, nor knowledge just for the learning, nor conflict just for the struggle. You see I finally realize this, and it seems so strange to me that so many people have not understood it yet.

A Polish gentleman was telling me today, "Life should have meaning. I find that philosophy is its highest expression. Philosophy should be the leader of every enlightened person."

"Alas," I answered him, "woe unto the man who surrenders to that blind woman to be led by her. The results will be his ruin. The true guide of a man's destiny is his own intuition because that springs from our inner source, while our thoughts are governed by all the outer influences. Any book you read, any person you speak with, will give you a different direction, a different conception of life. While our intuition springs from our needs, it is a gift with which nature has endowed man so that he may safely find his way, as the animals with their instinct."

"Nevertheless," he said to me, "I love philosophy and I shall leave experimental zoology to become a philosopher."

"Do you remember our friend, Krakowitz, in Trieste? He, too, has left zoology and is not a lecturer of philosophy in the University of Krakovia. The same with Driesch – from zoology, he is now a professor of philosophy at the University of Heidelberg."

"If you plan to be a philosopher like Driesch," I said to him, "it's best not to. Maybe he has a strong mind, but he has no conscience, as all metaphysicists. If in the end you become a philosopher, be careful not to leave the solid ground of reality and don't teach illusions for scientific facts. And most important of all, leave life alone and don't give her any idealogical content – be careful not to poison others. We two are poisoned enough."

My friend, Stangpwitz, looked at me confused, I was speaking in this manner – I, who when we were in Trieste, was full of idealism. Yes, one and the same. The only difference is that I have changed the color of my glasses with which I look at life. Now I don't see life as red or green or blue, nor anything like that, but white, only snow white, as she really is. Now I love her. I want to enjoy it.

I made a mistake to bring my books from Monaco. It is eleven o'clock and I have no time now for study. I worked enough all day. I am satisfied because I found something positive and I believe that very soon I can complete my work here.

I shall be very happy to return, for in spite of the reverence and admiration that I feel for this place, my soul is there with all of you. And I would be denying myself if I would think of giving sovereignity to the spirit and not to the emotion, but there is no such fear and the last of these is so beloved to me that nothing is capable of erasing this love.

Downstairs they're still dancing. The vibrations reach me up here. Oh, I am so grateful to them for the pleasure they have given me.

Nina, kiss all of them for me and many warm kisses and much love from your brother.

George

Back in Greece, ominous signs of war with Turkey reappeared and Dr. Papanicolaou was called into the army once more. On October 15, 1912, Greece joined the Balkan Alliance in war against Turkey. On the 9th of November, the Turkish Army in Salonika capitulated. The Greeks, who had been accused of contributing little to this victory, were determined to take Jenina by storm and continued further toward Turkey. However, by May 30, 1913, peace preliminaries with Turkey were agreed upon and signed. The peace preliminaries signed in London were never formalized, for war broke out between the Balkan allies. On June 29, the Bulgarians ordered a general attack on the Serbians and Greeks. This phase of the war was short lived, and an armistice between Bulgaria and the Greco-Serbian combination was signed. It became effective on August 1. The treaty of Bucharest on August 7, 1913, ended the war between Bulgaria and Greece.

Papanicolaou was promoted later to Lieutenant, Medical. He wrote little of his experiences in the Balkan War, but stated that he saw many horrors that such a war always involved. When George had entered the army, Mary remained in Kymi with his family. She spent her time both at her father-in-law's home and the home of her sister-in-law, Helen, who was married and lived a short distance away. She traveled by means of a horse- or donkey-drawn cart, the common conveyance at that time. When a cease-fire had been consummated between the warring forces,

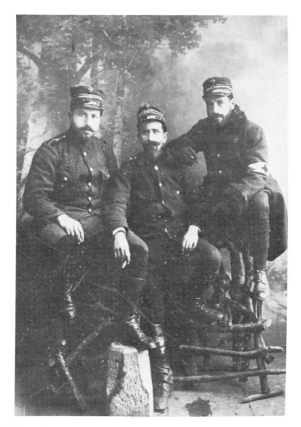

Figure 18. Papanicolaou and friends during the Balkan War, 1912-1913. Papanicolaou far right.

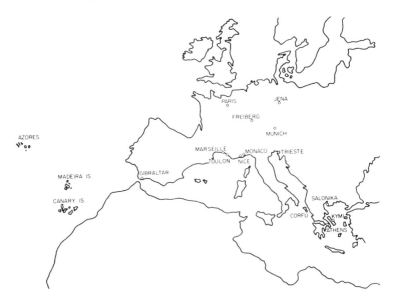

Figure 19.

arrangements were made for Mary to leave Kymi and proceed to Kozani in Macedonia to join her husband. This was accomplished by her father, Col. Mavroyeni, and she traveled in a military bus in the charge of officers, friends of her father. The couple remained in Kozani, a small town near Salonika, for approximately two months, extending to almost the time of Dr. Papanicolaou's discharge from military service. Mary returned to Athens to await her husband. When Dr. Papanicolaou returned, he confronted his father with news that he wished to migrate to America. During his military service he had come in contact with a number of Greek-American soldiers who told him of the opportunities in the United States. Dr. Nicholas was quite upset and said that his son would only be an immigrant, living among strangers away from family and friends. In spite of the many objections registered by both families, the young couple was determined to come to America. Dr. Papanicolaou, in order to allay the anxiety of his father, misinformed him by stating that he had obtained an offer for a job in America.

They obtained tickets for passage on the ship, Athenai. This was the same vessel which had taken them on their honeymoon cruise to Marseilles. Again Col. Mavroyeni paid for their first class passage. The couple had in cash only slightly more than $250, the amount required to enter the United States. They arrived in New York on October 19, 1913.

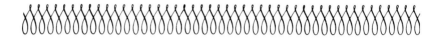

CHAPTER VI

EARLY YEARS IN
THE UNITED STATES

LEAVING family and familiar surroundings in exchange for a foreign country, without friends or established employment, was no easy matter. And without money there was no turning back at least for several years. What made matters worse, both families had bitterly objected to the decision. After the patience and support of their families through the troublesome and uncertain years, it was difficult to deny them their wish in their older, lonelier days. But the opportunity for a young research-oriented zoologist seemed better in America than in either impoverished, politically torn Greece or the strongly competitive and nationalistically oriented Germany. The new language would soon be no problem, but how could a foreigner obtain an academic position without established credentials and friends? There was one man who might help. Dr. T. H. Morgan of Columbia University had just published a book entitled HEREDITY AND SEX. Included in this volume were two pages which dealt with the experimental work presented by Papanicolaou in his Ph.D. thesis published in *Biologisches Centralblatt.* Dr. Morgan might have a research position available. If not, he would certainly know the availability of such positions in New York.

Hoping to find someone able to converse in Greek and give advice concerning their pressing need for employment, the Papanicolaous proceeded immediately to the Athens Hotel on 42nd Street after leaving the immigration station. Dr. Papanicolaou then contacted Dr. Morgan who insisted on giving a cocktail party for his foreign guest. Several well-known scientists from New York attended the party. Being too embarrassed to discuss employment with Dr. Morgan after this unexpected reception, the young zoologist applied for a job at Gimbel's Department Store.

Mary had just obtained a position there. She sewed buttons on altered garments for five dollars weekly. A French lady already working in this position had applied for a raise. After Mrs. Papanicolaou had shown great diligence and proficiency in this work, the French lady was fired and all the responsibility for such alterations was given to Mrs. Papanicolaou. It was especially difficult for her, however, since she understood and spoke little English at this time. She used to come home and cry because of so much work and such a communication problem.

Dr. Papanicolaou was also successful in obtaining employment at Gimbel's, but on his second day, while working as a rug salesman, he was asked to show a rug to a potential customer. The lady happened to be an acquaintance whom the young couple had met during their first class passage to the United States. So chagrined was he that this woman should see him selling rugs, he quit his job and returned to Dr. Morgan for help.

Dr. T. H. Morgan, one of the most widely known (Drosophila studies) and respected zoologists in America, was successful in obtaining for Papanicolaou a part-time position as assistant in the Department of Pathology and Bacteriology of the New York Hospital, then located on East 16th Street. The work was entirely technical and involved no research. After several months, during which time the job became full-time employment at sixty dollars monthly, Dr. William Elser recognized the superior ability and initiative of his new assistant. He suggested that Dr. Charles Stockard, Chairman of the Department of Anatomy of Cornell Medical College, might have a position available involving more challenging work. As a result of this excellent recommendation, Dr. Papanicolaou came to Cornell Medical School in September 1914. He received an increased income as assistant in the Department of Anatomy.

With this new assignment, he was able to give up his association with the Greek newspaper, *Atlantis,* which had employed him to write zoological tracts. After two months Mrs. Papanicolaou was also given a job in the Anatomy Department of Cornell University. She served as her husband's technician. Thus was formed a

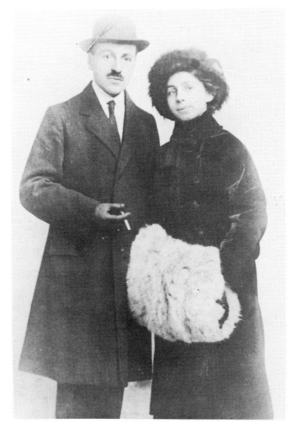

Figure 20. Mary and George Papanicolaou shortly after arrival in USA in 1913.

research team which would bear much fruit during the following half century.

Having rented an apartment on 27th Street and Lexington Avenue, just two blocks from Cornell Medical College, they lived within easy access to their research laboratory. After subletting one of the two bedrooms to a nurse, their seventy-five dollar monthly rental was reduced to a point which allowed them to save a small amount each month. But the most pleasing aspect of their new employment was the fact they were involved in research, with facilities and time to work independently along with their assigned project.

Dr. Stockard was an experimental anatomist, but his education and primary interest were in biology. He was a man of exceptional ability, combining an unusual originality and breadth of vision in his approach to problems. He was a highly disciplined personality, reminiscent of his earlier positions as Acting Professor of Military Science at Mississippi A & M College and later at Jefferson Military College. Dr. Stockard returned from work at the Zoological Station in Naples in 1911 to assume the Directorship of the Department of Anatomy at Cornell.

When Dr. Papanicolaou joined Dr. Stockard, Dr. Stockard was engaged in a series of experiments concerning the influence of alcohol on chromosomes and the transmission to progeny of any defects produced. Occurring just prior to prohibition, this subject had great popular appeal. As Dr. Papanicolaou was working with a large number of guinea pigs, he decided to continue his studies in sex determination which he had begun in Munich. In March 1915, he published his first American work in the periodical, *Science,* under the title "Sex Determination and Sex Control in Guinea Pigs." He suggested a transmissible sex tendency in both guinea pig parents, and a third sex determining factor which involved the parity of the mother. During the following year, two papers concerning the hereditary transmission of degeneracy and deformities in the descendants of the alcoholized animals were presented.

Interested in continuing his work on sex determination, Dr. Papanicolaou stated, "I asked for the privilege of using some animals in order to test the theory of sex determination by X and Y chromosomes in spermatozoa and ova." The experiments which he had in mind required obtaining the ova of the female guinea pigs at a precise stage of development. It was necessary to obtain the ova while they were undergoing mitotic division with the formation of polar bodies, approximately at maturity but before the extrusion of the ova from the follicles. He knew that this stage of development occurred at about the time of ovulation. As their work proceeded with the guinea pigs, it became more and more evident that the existing notions of the period of ovulation in the guinea pig were of no practical value, or were actually incorrect. Apparent solutions to this problem were most unsatisfactory, as they involved either the removal of the ovary by operation, or sacrificing the animal. In either case such a procedure would bring to conclusion the observations or experiments on the ovulation cycles in that particular animal.

Being thoughtfully bothered by this problem, he awoke one morning with the answer. Putting his thoughts on paper, he said, "The female of all higher animals have a periodic vaginal menstrual discharge; so lower animals, such as the rodent, should also have one but one probably too scanty to be evident externally." Recognizing that no thorough investigation of the uterus and vagina in the living female guinea pig had been made, it occurred to him that possibly estrous changes might take place, even though they were so feebly expressed as not to be noticeable on casual observation. The absence of an apparent estrous or proestrous flow from the vagina of the guinea pig had, as he stated, no doubt been the chief reason for the general lack of knowledge of the estrous cycle. He, therefore, determined to make a minute examination of the contents of the vagina of a number of virginal females every day for a long period of time, to ascertain whether a meager flow might exist, although insufficient in quantity to be noticed at the vaginal orifice or on the vulva.

On the way to Cornell Medical College that morning, Dr. Papanicolaou stopped at Tiemann's Surgical Supply Store and bought a small nasal speculum, which he planned to introduce into the vagina of each guinea pig utilized, for daily observation of the vaginal discharge. Later he decided in addition to take vaginal smears so that microscopic changes could also be assessed. Indeed he found in this animal a striking regularity of the "menstrual period," lasting 24 hours and recurring every 15 or 16 days. During this 24-hour "period," a characteristic fluid appeared which occasionally showed a slight trace of blood terminally but was usually milky white. "There were moments of real excitement when the examination of the first slides revealed an impressive wealth of diverse cell forms and a sequence of distinctive cytologic patterns."

The next task was to correlate the smear pattern with changes occurring in the uterus and ovary. When this was accomplished, it was possible to obtain the mature ova required for his research at precisely the right time.

The results of these correlative studies were first described and published in *Science,* July 1917. This report was followed in September of that year with a more detailed analysis of the subject which appeared under the authorship of Stockard and Papanicolaou in the *American Journal of Anatomy,* September 1917.

The great advantage of this simple method of examination for determining the estrous cycle in mammals which showed no external signs of heat, was evident to other zoologists immediately, and congratulations were extended to Dr. Stockard, who at that time was terminating his summer investigations in the Marine Biological Laboratory at Woods Hole, Massachusetts. After learning that Dr. Stockard had received all the credit for the experimental work on the estrous cycle of the guinea pig, Dr. Papanicolaou was very upset, contending that he would never be able to receive credit for his work as long as he was required to place the name of his chairman first in each paper. He considered employment elsewhere but decided to talk first with Dr. Stockard about this matter. Dr. Stockard appreciated the concern of his colleague and assured him that his name would never again have to be attached to work performed by Dr. Papanicolaou. This confirms the assessment made concerning Dr. Stockard by other associates who stated, "His consideration for the independence of and interest in the development of his colleagues and graduate students instill the deepest loyalty and cooperation."

The vaginal smear, as perfected in the course of these studies, soon found general application. The sex cycle of other rodents, such as the mouse and the rat, and of several higher mammals, such as the oppossum, sow and monkey, were studied and more minutely analyzed with the aid of this particular technique.

Drs. Evans and Long at Berkeley had been working on the ovulatory cycles of white mice. Since these mice ovulated 24 hours after they gave birth, an electronic monitoring device to alert the investigator was rigged such that just after birth the young mice would roll down the cage floor onto the electronic pad, tripping an alert signal, so that the investigator would not have to stay up all night waiting for this event. After reading the

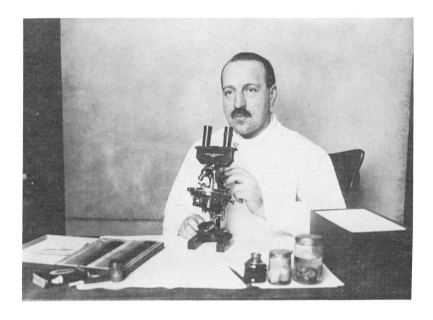

Figure 21. Papanicolaou, around 1919, examining guinea pig specimens at the New York Hospital.

THE EXISTENCE OF A TYPICAL OESTROUS CYCLE
IN THE GUINEA-PIG—WITH A STUDY OF ITS HIS-
TOLOGICAL AND PHYSIOLOGICAL CHANGES

CHARLES R. STOCKARD AND GEORGE N. PAPANICOLAOU

Department of Anatomy, Cornell University Medical School, New York City

ONE TEXT FIGURE AND NINE PLATES

1. INTRODUCTION

The existence of a more or less regular and definite oestrous cycle has been recognized in a number of mammals, particularly among the different classes of primates, carnivores, ungulates and insectivores. Yet very little is actually known or understood regarding the oestrous cycles and heat periods of a great many other very common mammals. Strangely enough, our knowledge of the sexual rhythm in the guinea-pig is much confused and not properly understood despite the great number of breeding experiments and the several studies of the sexual conditions which have been performed on this animal.

While conducting an extensive breeding experiment with guinea-pigs for the past several years it has become more and more desirable to know their exact oestrous periods.[1] A careful study of the existing literature bearing on this subject serves merely to produce uncertainty and confusion regarding their

[1] Throughout this paper we have used the terminology proposed by Heape, Quar. Jour. Mic. Sc., vol. 44, 1900, and adopted by Marshall and others. Anoestrous period or anoestrum, period of rest in the female; prooestrum, the first part of the sexual season; oestrus or oestrum, especial period of desire in the female; metoestrum, the short period when the activity of the generative system subsides and the normal condition is resumed in case conception did not occur; dioestrum, the short period of rest which in some mammals lasts only a few days. Such a short cycle as we shall describe in the guinea-pig consisting of four periods the prooestrum, oestrum, metoestrum and dioestrum is known as a dioestrous cycle.

Figure 22. Classical paper by Papanicolaou and Stockard which stimulated further research in cytology both in the human and other animal species.

article by Stockard and Papanicolaou, Long and Evans initiated studies on the sexual cycles of the rat utilizing vaginal cytology. "As the study progressed," according to Dr. George Corner, "their excitement became so great that they could hardly bear to leave the laboratory at the end of the day." After long hours of repeated observations, they were able to compile their monograph on the estrous cycle of the rat. The precision and scope of their own research was greatly facilitated by monitoring the periodic changes in the vaginal smear.

Establishment of a regular sex cycle in the guinea pig, mouse and rat proved to be of immense value in investigations and experimental studies on the reproductive tract. It also opened the way for new and significant observations and discoveries in biochemistry of sex hormones. Some years later in 1922, Edgar Allen recalled the Long-Evans monograph on the vaginal smear in the mouse. According to Dr. Corner, "Inevitably, however, with increasing knowledge of the mouse cycle, he was struck by the recurrent presence of large follicles just at the time of estrous . . ."* Like Marshall, 17 years before, Allen began to suspect that ovarian follicles produced an estrous hormone. He had, however, a much more practical and far more rapid test (i.e., the vaginal smear) for the presence of an estrous producing substance than Marshall, who had to watch for the slow onset of ill–defined signs of estrous in the dog. Allen, using the rat in place of the dog and applying the vaginal smear technique, could read the results of his tests in a day or two. With inspired simplicity, he collected follicle fluid from the sow's ovary and injected it into spayed mice. Within a few hours, the vagina began to show cytological changes characteristic of the estrous phase of the cycle and the animal shortly exhibited estrous behavior. This led to the detection of the ovarian estrogenic hormones by Allen and Doisy in 1923. Detection of the presence of estrogen by the vaginal smear also greatly facilitated the research of other investigators.

Prior to the isolation of the luteal hormones, Papanicolaou observed that injection of an extract of human luteal tissue into intact animals produced a cessation of cyclical changes in the

---

*Corner, George W.: The early history of the oestrogenic hormones. *Journal of Endocrinology, 31:*13, 1965.

vaginal smears. This he correlated with a pseudo-pregnancy state in the uterus and regression of the follicle in the ovary. The smears remained monotonous until the injections were stopped and then the cycles resumed. Soon afterwards, largely through Corner's important contributions, the luteal hormone was isolated.

Dr. Corner states, "In conjunction with the growing knowledge of the cycle of the sow and of reproduction in the rabbit, the vaginal smear method led indirectly to the discovery of the corpus luteum hormones and to a far clearer general comprehension of the whole field than was possible before."* For years the meeting of the American Society of Anatomists were virtually dominated by reports of work with the new vaginal smear technique.

However, amid his professional success there was sadness, for in 1919 Dr. Papanicolaou had been notified of the death of his father. Although his father had been extremely disappointed and felt that his son would be a failure in his new endeavor, neverthelsss some of the profound disappointment and sorrow initially evoked had subsided. Dr. Papanicolaou had corresponded with his father, but infrequently. His father's death in 1919, as well as the premature death of his sister, Helen, a few years prior, had been matters of grief and frustration to the scientist, since he was in a distant land and was unable to be present during these crucial family events.

In 1921 Dr. Papanicoalou had again been saddened through the temporary loss of an admired associate, Mr. Hashime Murayama. Mr. Murayama, who had been involved in the very delicate work of mounting and staining serial sections of the central nervous system for the Department of Anatomy, accepted an opportunity for employment by the National Geographic Society in Washington as an illustrator for their magazine. At Cornell he had occupied a room which adjoined that of Dr. Papanicolaou and they saw each other daily. So much did the scientist admire his friend that he praised him as exemplifying "the highest human qualities." Their paths were destined to cross years later in a celebrated collaborative effort.

In the early 1920's, during his second term as Premier of

---

*Corner, George W.: The Hormones in Human Reproduction. 1947, p. 73.

Greece, Venizelos had become aware of Papanicolaou's work and offered him an appointment as Professor of Zoology at the University of Athens. Dr. Papanicolaou had been reluctant to entertain the idea of moving from his laboratory at that time but communicated with the Premier on the matter. Then Premier Venezelos lost political favor and apparently concomitantly the effort for recruitment terminated. This had been the only consideration to return to Europe which Papanicolaou entertained for fifty years. His work had become established and a promising future seemed assured in his adopted country.

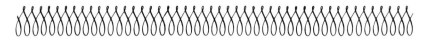

CHAPTER VII

DIAGNOSIS BY THE VAGINAL SMEAR

T HE new vistas opened to research by the cytological smear caused Papanicolaou to turn from his investigation of
the sex chromosomes to a comprehensive evaluation of the vaginal
smear. Having worked out the details of vaginal cytology in the
female guinea pigs, Dr. Papanicoloau recognized the possibility of
clinical use of this method in the human female. Meticulous
evaluation would be necessary, however, for it had already been
shown that cytological changes varied among different mammals.
Dr. Papanicolaou had begun his study of the vaginal cytology of
the human in 1920, using a special case which he continued to
study through 21 years. He stated that this was an ideal case
because of the perfect regularity in her menstrual periods and the
complete lack of any serious disturbance or any bacterial
contamination. This "special" case was later known to be that of
Mrs. Papanicolaou.

The application of vaginal cytology to women was somewhat
more difficult because the cytologic changes of the vaginal fluid
was less typically expressed than in some of the other mammals.
For this reason, most investigators who studied the problem had
generally reported unsatisfactory results. One might recall the
work of Pouchet, who in 1847 gave a description of human vaginal
smears and was able to recognize the existence of a rhythmical
change in the vaginal secretions. His work, however, was largely
lost sight of and in no way directed attention to the value of
vaginal cytology as an indicator of the phases of the sexual cycle.

Lehmann, in 1921, reported a study on the diagnostic value of
the human vaginal smear. He was interested chiefly from a
pathological and diagnostic point of view and did not attempt to
establish a definite morphological and physiological relationship
between the changes in vaginal fluid and the ovarian uterine cycle.

Many investigators were interested in the value of cytology as it pertains to women, but Allen expressed the prevailing opinion when he stated in 1925, "The smear test is of greatest value in animals in which sexual changes are not as clearly marked externally. In the primates, including women, menstruation furnished such a prominent milestone that vaginal smears seem of secondary importance for diagnosis."*

From 1920 until 1925, Dr. Papanicolaou's experience with vaginal cytology in women consisted primarily of the single "special" case. Vaginal smears were obtained during this time also from the clinic of Cornell Medical College and these were taken primarily from pathological cases. It now became clear that work should be done in an effort to assess the diagnostic capabilities, as well as to confirm further the normal baseline criteria for cytological changes in the human vagina.

In February of 1925, a valuable association was established between the Woman's Hospital of the City of New York and the Department of Anatomy at Cornell Medical College. Dr. George Gray Ward, Director of Woman's Hospital, was also Professor of Gynecology at Cornell Medical College and was responsible for the Cornell medical student program in gynecology. Dr. Papanicolaou, not being a clinician, had been unable to obtain a sufficient number of subjects for the study of cytology in women. It was his plan to delineate the cyclic cytologic changes in the vagina of women just as he had done with the female guinea pig. Dr. Stockard arranged with Dr. Ward, through a grant administered by the Committee on Problems of Sex of the National Research Council, in conjunction with Dr. Robert L. Dickinson, representing the Maternal Health Committee, to allow Dr. Papanicolaou to establish a project for the study of vaginal cytology of women.

Beginning on February 9, 1925, Dr. Papanicolaou engaged twelve selected cases, principally from personnel of the hospital, from whom he would obtain daily smears (except for holidays) for two to three months.

He was particularly interested in correlating the vaginal

---

*Allen, Edgar: Abstract on discussion on ovarian follicular hormone. *Journal of American Medical Association, 85:*405, 1925.

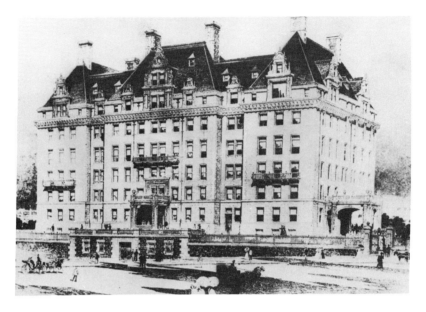

Figure 23. Woman's Hospital, New York City, 110th Street and Amsterdam
Avenue, where Papanicolaou performed first large-scale studies of human
vaginal cytology.

cytologic changes with ovarian and uterine physiology. For these
observations, he followed to the operating room certain patients
from whom he obtained preoperative vaginal smears.

In addition to these patients, he took serial vaginal smears from
pregnant women. After several months, he submitted his first
paper concerning human vaginal smears entitled "Human Pregnancy Diagnosis by Vaginal Smear."

After becoming thoroughly familiar with the normal cytologic
changes, Dr. Papanicolaou included pathologic cases in his study.
It was inevitable that among the pathologic cases which he
examined, some would have a genital malignancy. He has
remarked, "The first observation of cancer cells in a smear of the
uterine cervix was one of the most thrilling experiences of my
scientific career." He pursued an investigation of women with
genital malignancy and presented the results of this work with
cancer cytology at the Proceedings of the Third Race Betterment
Conference, which took place in Battle Creek, Michigan, in

January 1928. The title of the paper was "New Cancer Diagnosis." A newspaper article covering this meeting appeared in the *New York World* on January 5, 1928, and stated, "Although Dr. Papanicoloau is not willing to predict how useful the new diagnostic method will be in the actual treatment of malignancy itself, it seems probable that it will prove valuable in determining cancer in the early stages of its growth when it can be more easily fought and treated. There is even hope that pre-cancerous conditions may be detected and checked."*

The exact date of Dr. Papanicolaou's observation of cancer cells in a smear has not been determined. Whether he observed cancer cells in the several smears examined from the clinic at Cornell Medical College is not known. Dr. Papanicoloau, during later interviews, indicated that the association with Woman's Hospital occurred in 1923 which would suggest an earlier date for his initial work in cancer cytology. However, his papers published on the work which took place during this association state the "spring of 1925" as the beginning of this collaborative effort between the two institutions.

The fact that the cancer cytologic work was initially done at the Woman's Hospital is interesting. For it was a dispute with the lay board of Woman's Hospital concerning whether cancer patients should be admitted to the hospital which finally caused the famous founder of the hospital, Dr. Marion Sims, to resign. Dr.

---

*It is interesting to mention here the work of Dr. Aurel Babes, a Roumanian pathologist. In 1927 he collaborated with Dr. C. Daniel in presenting before the Society of Gynecology of Bucharest, two papers which proposed that human cervical cancer could be diagnosed by vaginal smear. The first paper involved six cases, to which were added several additional cases in the second paper. Four months after Papanicolaou reported his "New Cancer Diagnosis," Babes published in *La Presse Medicale* an article in which he suggested that an incipient stage of cervical carcinoma could be detected by vaginal smear.

As mentioned earlier, Papanicolaou had also conceived of this possibility. Just how early he had begun his work with the vaginal smear in cancer detection has not been clearly defined. However, several articles place the date as early as 1923 (1, 2, 3, 4).

1. Flach, Frederic F.: George Nicholas Papanicolaou. Cornell Medical Journal. December, 1948, p. 404.
2. Pierson, B.: *George N. Papanicolaou.*
3. Berkow, Samuel G.: After office hours, a visit with Dr. George N. Papanicolaou. *Obstetrics and Gynecology, 16*(no. 2)247, 1960.
4. Allegretti, Esther: *Cancer News,* 1957, p. 14.

NEW CANCER DIAGNOSIS

DR. GEORGE N. PAPANICOLAOU, Cornell University Medical College.

I will only give a report óf some work of mine which may have some bearing on the diagnosis of certain malignant tumors, especially those of the female genital tract.

This work was started about two and one-half years ago in the spring of 1925, first in the clinic of Cornell Medical College, then in the Women's Hospital in New York City. First we selected a number of normal women, and we took vaginal smears every day. The technique was very simple. We used a small pipette and took a little fluid from the vagina every day. Our intention was to find out if there was any definite morphological change in the vagina and the vaginal smear that would reveal some of the more important changes that occur in the ovaries and in the uterus.

As you probably know, this method has been applied very successfully in other mammals, especially in the rodents, with really surprising results. It has been possible to diagnose or to recognize certain changes in the ovaries and in the uterus. For instance, the time of ovalescence in the ovary may be ascertained by simply taking a little fluid from the vagina and examining it under the microscope. It would be ideal if we could apply this same simple method in human physiology and if we could, by the story of the vaginal smear, predict the condition of the ovary or of the uterus at a certain definite time. Unfortunately, the organ in the woman is a little more complex than it is in most other mammals, especially in the rodent; some of the typical changes in stages that occur in the organs that allow the recognition of corresponding changes in the ovary are not easily expressed. For instance, the beautiful leukocytic reaction in the rodents that characterizes certain stages and permits the diagnosis of ovarian and uterine changes are not so well expressed in the human. For this reason most investigators who had studied this problem did not report very satisfactory results. I am sorry I cannot report to you about these findings today because of limiting my presentation to the possible diagnosing of certain conditions, especially malignancy. Another factor that makes this work a little more difficult in the human is the tremendous variety of bacterial forms that are present in the human vagina; the number is much higher than that of/the bacterial flora in other mammals. In fact, in every case you may see very different flora, and this may be associated with various morphological conditions.

528

Figure 24. Papanicoalaou's "preliminary" findings on cancer cytology, published in 1928.

SDAY, JANUARY 5, 1928.

FINDS NEW CANCER DETECTION METHOD

New York Doctor Shows That Wounded Cells Elsewhere in Body Are Symptoms

"CANCER CAN BE BRED OUT"

Sterilization of Criminals Is Urged by Detroit Official

Science Service Special to The World

BATTLE CREEK, Mich., Jan. 4.—Discovery of a new method of diagnosing certain kinds of human cancers was announced to the Race Betterment Conference here to-day by Dr. George N. Pápanicolaou of Cornell Medical College, New York City.

Presence of cancer or malignant tumor is indicated by the changed forms of the cells and white corpuscles of the fluid in certain parts of the body away from the actual location of the cancerous growth. Under the microscope healthy cells and those that have been injured in the fight against cancer can be distinguished.

Although Dr. Papanicolaou is not willing to predict how useful the new diagnostic method will be in the actual treatment of malignancy itself, it seems probable that it will prove valuable in determining cancer in the early stages of its growth when it can be most easily fought and treated. There is even hope that pre-cancerous conditions may be detected and checked.

Figure 25. Newspaper article published by the New York World following Papanicolaou's first presentation of the diagnosis of cancer by the vaginal smear. In this article it was suggested that precancerous lesions might be detected by the cytological method.

Sims had insisted that cancer patients be admitted. The lay board of the hospital maintained that cancer patients, being incurable, needlessly occupied beds which could otherwise be used for patients with curable diseases, and in addition, the stench associated with cancer victims made hospitalization for the other patients unpleasant. During this era, it was the feeling among many of the general public that cancer was hereditary or of venereal origin and contagious, thereby stigmatizing both its victim and her family. Hospitals generally would not admit such patients or permit cancer surgery, thereby relegating treatment, including surgery, to private homes.

This dispute with the lay board of Woman's Hospital ultimately led to the founding of the New York Cancer Hospital, forerunner of the Memorial Hospital for Cancer and Allied Diseases. John J. Astor, influenced by his wife and her cousin, Mrs. Cullum, both members of the board of Woman's Hospital, offered to give one hundred fifty thousand dollars for the construction of a separate pavilion at Woman's Hospital for use exclusively in the treatment of cancer. When the offer was turned down, Mrs. Astor, Mrs. Cullum and others, spurred by a letter from Dr. Sims, decided to organize a cancer hospital in New York City. Ironically, by the time of incorporation of the new hospital, Mrs. Cullum was suffering from cancer of the uterus and Mrs. Astor was ill with a disease which circumstantial evidence suggested was also cancer.

During the annual board meeting of 1874, which occurred at the time of this "cancer" dispute, the Rev. Henry Potter stated rather prophetically concerning Woman's Hospital, "This hospital exists for the treatment of the diseases of women. Might it not properly undertake to do something for the prevention of those diseases?"* Although this last question could have been answered in the affirmative in 1928, another fifteen years was to pass before the value of cancer cytology would be appreciated by the medical world.

Dr. Papanicolaou's initial announcement of the diagnosis of cancer from the vaginal smear was received with little enthusiasm. As he stated it, "A brief preliminary paper in 1928 failed to

---

*Marı, J. P.: *Pioneer Surgeons.* 1957, p. 42.

convince my colleagues of the practicability of this procedure."
The prevailing opinion as expressed by one of the outstanding
pathologists of that time was that since the uterine cervix was
accessible to diagnostic exploration by biopsy, which is a relatively
simple procedure, the use of the cytologic examination of vaginal
smears appeared to be superfluous.

CHAPTER VIII

ENDOCRINE CYTOLOGY

ON May 22, 1928, four months after presenting his report, "New Cancer Diagnosis," Dr. George Papanicolaou became a citizen of the United States. During the almost fifteen years of residence, he had been promoted from Instructor in Anatomy to Assistant Professor of Anatomy and had become widely known in biological circles.

Beginning with experimental work in guinea pigs, he had begun to realize that his cytological method held unlimited potential as a diagnostic tool. Due to species differences, it had also become apparent that the application of this method for the benefit of humans required human investigation rather than animal. Until 1925 he had been able to study in depth only his one "special" case. But after the doors of Woman's Hospital had been opened to him, an "opportunity to study a large number of human vaginal smears from normal cases, as well as from cases of pregnancy and from several pathological conditions," had been afforded. In order to correctly identify normal changes, it became obvious that he must recognize clearly pathological alterations. Thus, he collected smears from various abnormal conditions, including "inflammatory conditions of the vagina, of the uterus, of the tubes; cases of tubercle abscesses; cases of ovarian cysts and other conditions of the ovary; and also cases of pregnancy, including tubal pregnancies and abortions; and finally, cases of benign and malignant tumor."

The vaginal smear seemed to possess its greatest potential as a diagnostic tool for cancer detection and in reflecting the presence and interaction of hormones. In cases of inflammatory processes and benign tumors, the vaginal smear was less definitive in its application. As an aid in uterine cancer detection, he concluded by stating that "A better understanding and a more accurate analysis of the cancer problem is bound to result from the use of this method." Due to the lack of enthusiasm of his colleagues, however, he was to change the emphasis of his cytological research to endocrine problems, leaving the application of the momentous discoveries in cancer diagnosis for another decade.

"The Sexual Cycle in the Human Female" appeared in monograph length in *The American Journal of Anatomy* in 1933. It was a compendium of the normal cytological changes occurring in the reproductive cycle of the human female. These painstaking and meticulous analyses of cellular alterations attested to the long years of careful observation through the microscope. This report established human cytology on a firm basis.

Following this publication, Dr. Papanicolaou described the vaginal cytology of the newborn, the child, and the menopausal woman to extend his observations to include varying normal hormonal phases in the life of the human female. In addition, the effects of estrogen and androgen on the cytology of the castrated or menopausal woman and the woman with certain menstrual problems were evaluated. By this time, Cornell Medical College had moved to York Avenue and 68th Street in the new facilities for the New York Hospital – Cornell Medical Center.

In 1934 cooperative studies between Dr. Papanicolaou and Dr. Ephraim Shorr of the Department of Endocrinology at Cornell began. This association was to permit an application of the vaginal smear on a much larger scale in the field of human endocrinology than previously possible. The collaborators recognized the value of the vaginal smears as a biological assay for estrogen. Utilizing this method, they also noted the apparent neutralizing effect of androgen when given in conjunction with estrogen to the menopausal woman.

Dr. Papanicolaou made several observations concerning amenorrheic women, in that some showed an atrophic type of vaginal smear, indicating a castrate picture whereas others showed some cyclic cytological variation and still others demonstrated a moderate estrogen response. He also pointed out from his endocrine investigations that the degree of symptomatic improvement and the extent of change in the smear in cases of castrates or

THE SEXUAL CYCLE IN THE HUMAN FEMALE AS REVEALED BY VAGINAL SMEARS[1]

GEORGE N. PAPANICOLAOU
Department of Anatomy, Cornell University Medical College, and Woman's Hospital, New York City

THREE FIGURES AND TEN PLATES (EIGHTY-ONE FIGURES)

I. INTRODUCTION

The study of the female sexual functions in mammals has been greatly stimulated and advanced in recent years by the application of the vaginal smear method. This method, as originally applied to the guinea pig by Stockard and Papanicolaou in 1917, consists in the microscopic examination of smears prepared at frequent intervals from the fluid content of the vagina. The vaginal fluid usually has a mucous consistency and contains a variety of desquamated cells, as well as leucocytes, lymphocytes, often erythrocytes, and a large number of bacteria. As the relative number and the distribution of these elements change periodically, smears prepared from such fluid show modifications in their composition and structure. The successive alternation of periods of sexual activity and inactivity, which characterizes the mammals, imparts to the vaginal fluid a rhythmical sequence of typical cellular stages which can be easily recognized.

These cyclic changes affect the entire genital tract, and, consequently, every change in the vaginal fluid is strictly correlated with corresponding changes in the other organs of the female genital system, particularly the uterus and the ovaries. The time of ovulation may be accurately detected

[1] This work has been aided by the Committee for Research on Sex Problems of the National Research Council, and by the National Committee on Maternal Health.

519

THE AMERICAN JOURNAL OF ANATOMY, VOL. 52, NO. 3, SUPPLEMENT
MAY, 1933

Figure 26. Monograph-length paper summarizing the normal cytological findings in the vagina of the human female.

menopausal women were not necessarily correlated. In some patients, relief from the menopausal symptoms could be obtained through estrogen therapy with only a slight change occurring in the smear, while in others complete reversal of the smear was necessary.

The potency of estrogenic compounds was also evaluated by employing the cytological method. The tremendously increased potency of ethinyl estradiol when compared to stilbestrol was cited. It was postulated that differential rates of liver metabolism of synthetic and naturally occurring estrogens accounted for the apparent greater absorption of stilbestrol when compared to estrone. The smear technique offered rather conclusive evidence concerning the amount of hormone actually reaching the body tissues, so that patient error in medication or possibly an absorption problem could be detected. It was at this time also that nausea was found to be rather common with the synthetic estrogens, while the naturally occurring estrogens were noted to lack side-effects. Abnormal hormone variations, as demonstrated by vaginal smears, were reported in psychiatric patients, suggesting that certain physiological changes were associated with mental illness and warranted more detailed research.

Papanicolaou had formulated a cell-staining technique which provided sharp definition of the cell wall and the fine details of the cell nucleus. Experimentation with the staining technique for the smears continued with minor modifications being made. A more rapid technique with more definitive cytoplasmic staining was developed by Shorr, which seemed superior if the purpose of the smear was for hormonal evaluation only.

During this period of time, Dr. Papanicolaou had been able to continue his cytological research involving a variety of gynecological problems through the clinical help of Drs. Andrew Marchetti, Carl Javert and Ralph Benson of the Department of Obstetrics and Gynecology. As time passed, they also became quite proficient in cytological diagnosis.

Dr. Papanicolaou began to see private pateints in consultation. Infertility patients* were often referred to him for endocrine

*It is interesting that in 1933, while taking serial smears from a clinic infertility patient, Dr. Papanicolaou discovered an unsuspected intraepithelial carcinoma. The initial cervical biopsy was negative but a second one was positive.

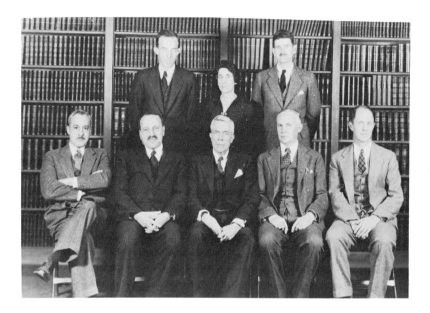

Figure 27. Department of Anatomy, Cornell Medical School, around 1936. Front row, l to r: Dr. J. Nonidez, Dr. Papanicolaou, Dr. C. Stockard, Dr. C. Morrell, Dr. P. Armstrong.

evaluation. One of his patients, the wife of a wealthy Greek businessman, later became pregnant. Through this limited private practice, the scientist was gradually able to accumulate enough money to more farther away from busy Manhattan.

Having moved to Long Island after the noise of the building of the subway had forced them to leave their apartment on 96th Street and Central Park West, the Papanicolaous bought a modest home in Douglaston in about 1927. Their happiest days were spent in Douglaston. In 1952 they moved to a larger home in Douglaston where Mrs. Papanicolaou had her beautiful garden and, being near the water, a varied scene for short walks was afforded. An upstairs room became the famous "study" where so much of the cytological work was performed. After dinner and a short period of relaxation with music and the newspaper, the scientist would continue his day's work in the quiet seclusion of this study. Mrs. Papanicolaou always made sure that orange juice was available at his desk and study would continue until about 1:00 A.M.

On occasion, especially the weekend, the Papanicolaous entertained friends. Mrs. J. F. Nonidez, wife of one of the scientist's early associates in the department of anatomy, remembers Dr. Papanicolaou as a genial host and recalls the twinkle in his eye as he related humorous incidents in his life. Home entertaining became more frequent as the years passed and were a source of great pleasure to the couple. However the guests, aware of his strict study schedule, were careful not to interfere too much with the established routine.

In 1939 Dr. Stockard died. The uncertainty which always accompanies a change in leadership followed. Dr. Stockard had continued his support of the work of Dr. Papanicolaou through the years, allowing him to spend almost all his time in research, rather than requiring of him a strict schedule of teaching responsibilities in the department. Dr. Stockard was succeeded by the able Dr. Joseph Hinsey who assumed the joint chairmanships of the Department of Anatomy and Physiology of the Cornell Medical Center.

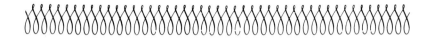

CHAPTER IX

THE PAP SMEAR

ONE of the first tasks confronting Dr. Hinsey as Chairman of the Department of Anatomy at Cornell was to learn his staff, their previous scientific contributions and their research interests for the future. By this time, Papanicolaou had terminated his cooperative studies with Dr. Epharim Shorr, but he had continued his work on the vaginal cytology of the guinea pig, especially the changes associated with senility. In addition, several research projects involving the sex hormones were in progress. However, the 1928 report, "New Cancer Diagnosis," had come to the attention of Dr. Hinsey. The idea intrigued him and he thought that it should be explored in more depth.

One day Dr. Papanicolaou came to Dr. Hinsey to obtain approval for a grant of about $4,000 from a pharmaceutical company for a project to determine the effect of androgen on muscle tissue. "He was somewhat taken aback when I urged him not to take it," recalls Dr. Hinsey, "but instead to devote all his time to developing his cytological method for diagnosis of early cancer in the reproductive tract of women." Dr. Papanicolaou expressed his previous discouragement and his anxiety concerning the availability of sufficient funds and clinical material for the task. Dr. Hinsey promised his wholehearted support and together they outlined a program whereby "the first step would be the development and the establishment of its validity; the second phase would be to train others to use it; and finally, an effort would be made to educate the medical profession and the public concerning what the method had to offer."

The plan was discussed with Dr. H. J. Stander, Chairman of the Department of Obstetrics and Gynecology. He encouraged Dr. H. F. Traut, gynecological pathologist on his staff, to work with Dr.

Papanicolaou. With the formation of this association and the financial support of the Department of Anatomy, the reevaluation of the vaginal smear for cancer detection was initiated in October 1939. All women admitted to the gynecological service of the New York Hospital were required to have a routine vaginal smear. A curved glass pipette with a strong rubber bulb for suction was used to obtain exfoliated cells from the posterior fornix of the vagina. A smear of the cellular contents of this aspirated material was then made on a glass slide and the specimen was immediately fixed in an ether-alcohol mixture.* Later the slides were stained† and then interpreted under the supervision of Dr. Papanicolaou. It soon became evident that "by use of the vaginal smear, a considerable number of asymptomatic and therefore unsuspected cases of uterine malignancy have been discovered, some of them in such an early stage of development that they were invisible to the unaided eye, or undemonstrable by the biopsy method," wrote Dr. Papanicolaou.

On March 11, 1941, a paper entitled, "The Diagnostic Value of Vaginal Smears in Carcinoma of the Uterus," was presented by Papanicolaou and Traut before the New York Obstetrical Society. Dr. I. C. Rubin terminated his comments on this presentation by stating, "If this proves diagnostic in a large number of cases of hidden type of carcinoma and of the early hitherto unrecognizable carcinoma of the cervix by the usual means at our disposal, including the colposcope, then we have made a great advance in the armamentarium in this field." And Dr. Hinsey was careful to observe that "this problem is different from tissue pathology. In tissue pathology we have not only the cytology of the cells involved, but also the orientation of those cells in the tissue. Here we are dealing primarily with the cytology of cells and are faced with problems which are like those of the hematologist who makes

---

*Papanicolaou initially used Carnoy's fixative consisting of absolute alcohol, chloroform and acetic acid for wet fixation but later deleted acetic acid, exchanged ether for chloroform because of the latter's distasteful odor and used 95% alcohol instead of absolute alcohol, which was difficult to procure.
†The wet-fixed slides were stained at first with hemotoxylin and eosin but when eosin alone was found to be an inadequate counterstain to produce clear differentiation between basophilic and acidophilic cells, a combination of eosin and Wasser Blau was utilized. Modifications after 1939 produced a three-step staining technique consisting of hematoxylin, followed by Orange G, then EA 36 which was composed of light green, bismarck brown and eosin.

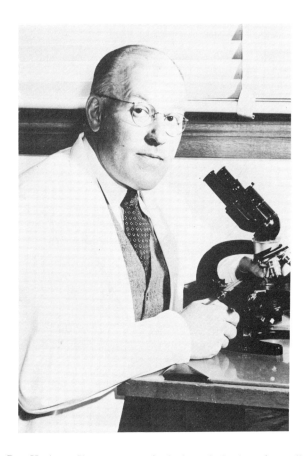

Figure 28. Dr. Herbert Traut, gynecological pathologist who collaborated with Papanicolaou in validating the diagnostic potential of the cancer smear.

his examination of the blood smear. The interpretations here have been possible only through the very broad and long study which Dr. Papanicolaou has made of the cytology of these cells in the female reproductive tract, combined with the knowledge of gynecologic pathology which Dr. Traut possesses."

This report was published in the *American Journal of Obstetrics and Gynecology* in August of that same year and constituted the fifty-sixth publication of Dr. Papanicolaou. At this time he was 58 years of age, but he was destined to triple this number of publications during the next 20 years.

The method was not ready for application on a large scale. In the 1941 report the authors had concluded "few persons can be depended upon for this work at the present time. However, if the method proves to be worthy of further development, as we expect it to be, then it will be possible, in a relatively short time, to provide the necessary facilities for instruction." They wanted to be sure beyond doubt that the smear technique was valid. Dr. Papanicolaou throughout his research career had rechecked his findings before allowing them to be published as fact. More data was necessary to establish absolutely the soundness of the method. This information continued to accumulate rapidly.

Following the publication in 1941, a grant of eighteen hundred dollars was made by the Commonwealth Fund to aid the work. The increased interest and generosity of this philanthropic organization permitted through the years the employment of additional personnel and the publication of classical monographs. Indeed, during the next decade their financial contributions amounted to one hundred twenty-four thousand dollars.

Among those who joined the team early was Mr. H. Murayama. After leaving the Cornell Anatomy Department in 1921, he had been continually employed by the National Geographic Society as a staff illustrator, specializing in watercolor paintings of fowl. Upon learning of his impending retirement, Dr. Papanicolaou wrote him of his exciting work with the cancer smear and his great need for an illustrator. So subtle were some of the important cytological alterations to which Dr. Papanicolaou and Dr. Traut wished to draw attention, that they felt only a skilled artist could present them properly. Mr. Murayama accepted the challenge and returned to New York.

Dr. A. Marchetti also became deeply involved in the work. He recalled that with the broad international involvement in the Second World War, a certain tenseness initially prevailed among the project staff. Dr. Traut, of Nordic ancestry, Dr. Marchetti, Italian, Mr. Murayama, Japanese, and Dr. Papanicolaou, Greek, in themselves represented several national interests. A closeness was reestablished among the staff, however, after a discussion was held wherein it was stated that "all were seeking the truth" and that national conflicts should not alter their personal friendships.

Apparently only because the war had detained a son of Mr. Murayama in Japan, the U. S. Government required Dr. Traut and Dr. Marchetti to be responsible for him.

As experience with the vaginal smear technique expanded, several interesting cases which emphasized the merits of this method were recorded. At the annual meeting of the Medical Society of the State of New York on April 30, 1942, two of these were presented. One was that of a 61-year-old lady who was referred to the gynecologist because of chronic bladder problems. A vaginal smear suspicious of malignancy was obtained but curettage and multiple cervical biopsies failed to disclose cancer. Finally after positive smears suggesting adenocarcinoma of the endometrium were repeatedly obtained during a four-month period and another curettage had produced only benign tissue, a third curettment was performed. A fragment of tissue from this procedure was read as benign by some pathologists and as probably malignant by others. After hysterectomy the uterus was found to contain a polypoid area of carcinoma located behind a small undetected leiomyoma in the left cornu.

A second case was referred to the gynecologist because of a "relaxed pelvic floor." The vaginal smear revealed cells that were thought to be characteristic of squamous cell carcinoma of the cervix. The most minute examination of the cervix and vagina failed to reveal any visible lesions. Repeated biopsies did not demonstrate a malignancy. The patient was kept under surveillance for four months. Then a small area of leukoplakic epithelium was observed and a biopsy was made. This specimen clearly showed an early squamous cell carcinoma of the cervix.

Two important points were made concerning the above cases: the vaginal smear permitted a diagnosis at a much earlier date than would have been possible by the biopsy technique and the diagnosis would not have been made had routine vaginal smears of all patients not been taken.

Such a wealth of confirmatory data was collected that Papanicolaou and Traut were confident of their findings and conclusions. Although Papanicolaou had planned to produce a monograph on the normal cytology of the female reproductive tract, he decided that the benefits to be derived from the large scale use of the cancer detection smear and the establishment of priority in the matter required that a monograph on this subject be published first.

The now famous and classic monograph, "Diagnosis of Uterine Cancer by the Vaginal Smear," was published by the Commonwealth Fund in 1943. Beside presenting the characteristics of normal and malignant cells found in vaginal smears and presenting illustrative case reports, the authors stressed that early noninvasive carcinomas could be discovered by the method and even suggested that women could be taught to obtain their own smears. Placed on sale for five dollars, it consisted of 61 pages of text with 22 pages of beautifully illustrated plates drawn by Mr. Murayama. Camera lucida sketches were made and colored while the artist reviewed the slide under the microscope. He performed his work so carefully that the relative sizes and shapes of the cells and their staining reactions were clearly recorded. In order to make the cilia and intercellular bridges distinct, the artist used a brush from which he pulled every bristle but one. The authors stated that "many characteristics of the cells would have gone unnoticed had it not been for the collaboration of Mr. Murayama." The technical aspects of the publication also received the untiring attention of Mrs. Papanicolaou and Miss Charlotte Street, Chief Cytological Technician. Mrs. Papanicolaou was now volunteering her services, as Dr. Hinsey had felt that it was inappropriate for husband and wife to be employed as staff on the same project. The Department of Gynecology gave its full support.

About the time the monograph appeared, the well-known and respected Dr. James Ewing, Director of Memorial Hospital for Cancer and Allied Diseases, died of urinary bladder cancer. During the decade following Dr. Papanicolaou's first announcement of a "new cancer diagnosis," Dr. Ewing had changed from his initial skepticism to a proponent of the method. In fact, five years before his death, he began to perform intermittent examinations of his urinary sediment following the removal of stones. As time passed, he happened to observe cancer cells. After cystoscopy revealed a fundal carcinoma of the bladder and an operation was performed, Dr. Ewing requested the slides for his examination. Hoping to keep the diagnosis from him, substitute slides were presented. To

DIAGNOSIS OF UTERINE CANCER
BY THE VAGINAL SMEAR

GEORGE N. PAPANICOLAOU, M.D., Ph.D.

Department of Anatomy, Cornell University Medical College

AND

HERBERT F. TRAUT, M.D.

Department of Obstetrics and Gynecology, Cornell University Medical College and the New York Hospital

NEW YORK: THE COMMONWEALTH FUND
1943

Figure 29. Title page of the Papanicolaou-Traut monograph on the canc smear.

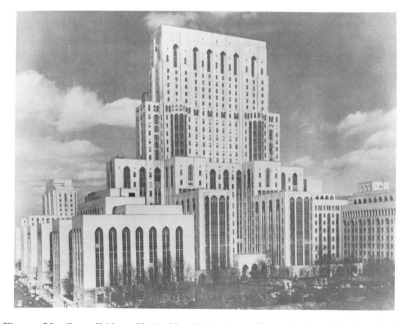

Figure 30. Cornell-New York Hospital where Papanicolaou developed the cancer (Pap) smear.

the surprise of those present, he announced that the slides were not his. "I have already seen the type of cell associated with my type of bladder cancer."*

The observations of Papanicolaou and Traut were soon confirmed by other investigators, including Meigs, Graham and Fremont-Smith in Boston and Neustaedter and Mackenzie in New York. The first phase of the initial plan (that of establishing validity of the method) had essentially been accomplished. However, the value of cytology in cancer detection was not accepted by most pathologists and several years would pass before this important step would be realized. The capability of detecting cancer of the cervix before invasion occurred had apparently not been fully appreciated, and even if the smear technique had the capability of such detection, the pathologist, it was said, would not have time to review the large number of slides necessary to find a positive case. The great Dr. Robert Meyer of Berlin, whose classic study in 1911 put the relationship between ovarian function and cyclic changes in the endometrium on a sound basis, seemed to share this opinion. He did not live to see the full development of the technique.

In 1945 great impetus was given to the movement to educate the profession concerning the value of the vaginal smear by the newly formed American Cancer Society. Actually, this organization was the outgrowth of the former American Society for the Control of Cancer, founded in 1913. This older organization had been created by several gynecologists and public-spirited laymen who wanted to impress women with the danger signs of uterine cancer, in an effort to treat cancer before it became advanced.

The recognition of the need for more research concerning cancer led the newly named American Cancer Society to reserve 25 percent of its funds for this purpose. At this same time, the Society was fortunate in choosing a man of unusual ability and energy, Dr. Charles Cameron, to serve as medical and scientific director. Through the effort of Dr. Cameron, The American Cancer Society sponsored the First National Cytology Conference in Boston in 1948. The conference was attended by more than

*Bamforth, J. and Osborn, G. R.: Diagnosis from cells. *Journal of Clinical Pathology* 11:478, 1958.

ninety persons with special interest in cytology. This group concluded that of all the procedures available, the vaginal smear was unique in that it was capable of detecting uterine cancer before it became visible to the naked eye and before it produced the danger signals of cancer. A note of warning was again voiced, very likely by Dr. Papanicolaou, that no intensive campaign should be conducted to bring large numbers of women to their physicians' offices until sufficient numbers of pathologists and technicians could be trained to interpret the smears correctly. The method might have suffered discredit had a tremendous wave of patient demand suddenly been imposed on the pathologists at large, many of whom at that time were unfamiliar with the cytologic interpretation. Dr. Papanicolaou credited Dr. Cameron with the foresight and careful planning which popularized the vaginal smear method in cancer diagnosis.*

In order to help relieve the manpower shortage, Dr. Papanicolaou organized and taught a course in cytology at the New York-Cornell Medical Center beginning in September 1947. Seventy participants, forty-five of whom were pathologists from various states in the nation, attended the first course. Many individuals had visited and received instruction in cytology in his laboratory prior to the establishment of this special course.

The monograph on "Epithelia of Woman's Reproductive Organs," the writing of which had been delayed in favor of the monograph on cancer, appeared in 1948. The publication was co-authored by Drs. Papanicolaou, Traut and Marchetti. By this time, Dr. Traut had accepted the chairmanship of the Department of Obstetrics and Gynecology at the University of California and Dr. Marchetti had assumed the chairmanship of the Department of Obstetrics and Gynecology at Georgetown Medical Center.

Carcinoma of the vagina, cervix, endometrium and fallopian tube had been diagnosed through vaginal and uterine aspiration

---

*Papanicolaou felt that there were two underlying scientific factors which were decisive in the ultimate acceptance of the "cancer smear." One factor was wet fixation (instead of air or heat fixation) of the smears which preserved the fine structural details of the cells. The other factor was the acquisition of a broad basic knowledge of the normal exfoliated cytology of the female genital tract which afforded comparison with the abnormal features of exfoliated malignant cells.

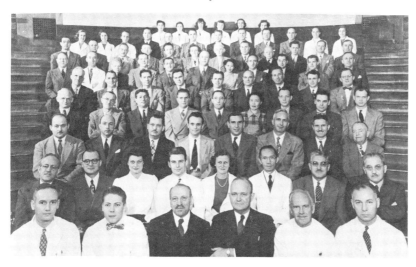

Figure 31. Front row, l to r: Dr. John Seybolt, Dr. Rogers, Dr. Papanicolaou, Dr. Joseph Hinsey, Dr. Foot and Dr. Terzano. Miss Charlotte Street and Mr. H. Murayama are sitting behind and just right of Dr. Papanicolaou.

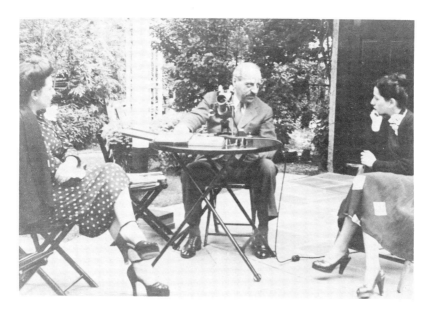

Figure 32. Papanicolaou at home in Douglaston, Long Island, New York. His typical glasses-on-forehead pose is shown here.

smears. Application of the smear technique for cancer detection also had been extended to urine, sputum, gastric washings, ascites, prostate secretions, spinal fluid and breast secretions. A renal carcinoma was found at surgery in a patient who consistently demonstrated malignant cells in the urine but who had no lesion otherwise demonstrable. A 50-year-old man with chronic bronchitis was found to have an abnormal smear on routine sputum examination. Clinical evaluation including x-rays and bronchoscopy were all negative for tumor. At autopsy, no tumor could be found in the bronchial tree or lungs. Random specimens of the bronchial mucosa, however, established the presence of carcinoma *insitu* at a point about 2 cm below the origin of the right lower bronchus. Dr. Emerson Day reported two cases from the Memorial Hospital for Cancer and Allied Diseases. One involved a 51-year-old lady who had recurrent "positive" vaginal smears but no lesion could be located. Hysterectomy was scheduled, but at the time of operation, a posterior vaginal carcinoma was found which necessitated radical surgery. Another patient at operation had an infiltrating ductal carcinoma of the breast after physical examination had failed to detect an abnormality suggested by "positive" cytology.

Dr. Day recalls the reaction of Dr. Papanicolaou to the unfruitful search for a lesion in one of these cases. "Dr. Papanicolaou became alarmed, declaring that if we were unable to confirm a positive diagnosis in this patient in face of such overwhelming cytologic evidence, the cytologic method might have to be abandoned."

Dr. Papanicolaou developed five categories of classification of vaginal smears: Class I – normal; Class II – inflammatory; Class III – suspicious for malignancy; Class IV – strongly suggestive of malignancy and Class V – definitely malignant. Relative to the latter classification, he stated in 1948, "there are, however, cases in which major operations have been performed on the strength of a positive Class V smear report prior to confirmation by biopsy. By being very conservative in our Class V reports, we have actually demonstrated that the smear method can be trusted as a method of final diagnosis."

Following the publication, "Epithelia of Woman's Reproductive

THE EPITHELIA OF
WOMAN'S REPRODUCTIVE ORGANS

A CORRELATIVE STUDY OF CYCLIC CHANGES

GEORGE N. PAPANICOLAOU, M.D., PH.D.
*Professor of Clinical Anatomy, Cornell
University Medical College*

HERBERT F. TRAUT, M.D.
*Professor of Obstetrics and Gynecology
University of California Medical School*

AND

ANDREW A. MARCHETTI, M.D.
*Associate Professor of Obstetrics and Gynecology
Cornell University Medical College*

NEW YORK: THE COMMONWEALTH FUND
1948

Figure 33. Title page of Papanicolaou's second monograph. It presented the normal cytology of the female reproductive tract.

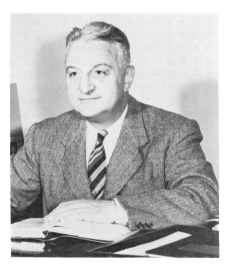 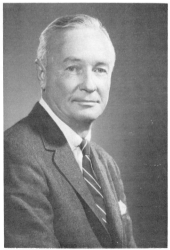

Figure 34. *(Left)* Andrew Marchetti who collaborated with Papanicolaou and Traut on the monograph "Epithelia of Woman's Reproductive Organs." *(Right)* Charles Cameron, friend and confidant; credited by Papanicolaou with popularizing the cancer smear.

CORNELL UNIVERSITY
MEDICAL COLLEGE

1300 YORK AVENUE
New York City

DEPARTMENT OF ANATOMY

October 18, 1948

Dr.
Room
The New York Hospital

Report on

Vaginal and cervical smears of 10/8/48:
Negative for neoplastic cells.
Menopausal type. Bacterial flora
of bacilli. Leucocytes on the
profuse side. One small polypoid
endocervical cell cluster in the
cervical smear indicating the
presence of some papillary growth
in the endocervical mucosa.

Class I.

George N. Papanicolaou
George N. Papanicolaou, M. D.

GNP/eca

CORNELL UNIVERSITY
MEDICAL COLLEGE

1300 YORK AVENUE
New York City

DEPARTMENT OF ANATOMY

May 29, 1950

Dr.

New York Hospital

Report on

Vaginal smears of 3/28/50. Negative
for neoplastic cells. Menopausal atrophic
cytology. Numerous leucocytes and histiocytes suggestive of a cervical infection.
Bacterial flora mixed.
            Some cells show slight atypia, but
not sufficient to arouse suspicion of
malignancy. Class II.

George N. Papanicolaou
George N. Papanicolaou, M.D.

GNP:jr

Figure 35. Class I and Class II Papanicolaou smear reports with benign findings.

CORNELL UNIVERSITY
MEDICAL COLLEGE
1300 YORK AVENUE
NEW YORK CITY

DEPARTMENT OF ANATOMY

January 24, 1951

Dr.

Report on

Cervical smears of 1-23-51. Many atypical cells characteristic of dyskaryosis mixed type, chiefly superficial and parabasal. It is likely that the patient has an early malignant cervical lesion, which is progressing slowly.

Class III.

George N. Papanicolaou

George N. Papanicolaou, M.D.

GNP/rab

CORNELL UNIVERSITY
MEDICAL COLLEGE
1300 YORK AVENUE
NEW YORK CITY

DEPARTMENT OF ANATOMY

January 22, 1953

Dr.

New York Hospital

Report on

Cervical smears of 1/21/53. Fairly conclusive evidence of an adenocarcinoma of the endometrium.

Class IV

G. Papanicolaou

George N. Papanicolaou, M.D.

GNP/ja

Figure 36. Class III and Class IV Papanicolaou smears suggestive of malignancy.

DEPARTMENT OF ANATOMY
CORNELL UNIVERSITY MEDICAL COLLEGE
1300 YORK AVENUE, NEW YORK CITY

PAPANICOLAOU RESEARCH LABORATORY

March 26, 1958

Dr.

Room

Report on

Vaginal and cervical smears of 3-25-58. Conclusive evidence of a malignant neoplasm. Type consistent with an adenocarcinoma.

Class V.

G. Papanicolaou

George N. Papanicolaou, M.D.

GNP:jf

CORNELL UNIVERSITY
MEDICAL COLLEGE
1300 YORK AVENUE
NEW YORK CITY

DEPARTMENT OF ANATOMY

April 9, 1952

Dr.

New York Hospital

Report

Endometrial smears of 4/7/52. Conclusive evidence of an adenocarcinoma of the endometrium with adenoacanthomatous areas. This appears to be a rather advanced infiltrating carcinoma.

Class V.

Note: The diagnosis is well enough established to justify a major operation without a curettage.

George N. Papanicolaou

George N. Papanicolaou, M.D.

GNP:mn

Figure 37. Class V smears. Dr. Papanicolaou was very conservative in designating a smear Class V, therefore he often felt that his Class V smears were diagnostic of malignancy.

Organs," Dr. Papanicolaou began his monumental task of preparing the comprehensive "Atlas of Exfoliative Cytology." This manual included a review of the cytology of all regions subjected to study. In addition to Mr. Murayama's drawings, it would include color photomicrographs. The job was finally completed in 1954. Produced in loose-leaf form, it was planned that new information might be easily added to keep the text always current.

That same year, the American Cancer Society discussed the tremendous potentialities of exfoliative cytology. Pilot projects for mass cytologic screening had been initiated to determine the effectiveness of the "Pap" smear from an epidemiological standpoint.* The ability of trained technicians to accurately screen the large number of routine smears had been proven, vindicating Dr. Papanicoloau's pleas of the previous decade. The national press published reports on the merits of the cancer smear and the American Cancer Society continued to wage its campaign of educating the public. And the public was becoming more aware. The program conceived fifteen years before was now entering its final phase. A milestone had been reached in the life of the scientist, now a clinical professor of anatomy.

*One of the earliest and largest of these surveys involved 95,000 women located in the Memphis, Tennessee area. The National Cancer Institute sponsored this project.

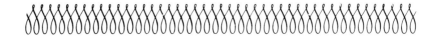

CHAPTER X

DREAMS FULFILLED

IN a letter to Dr. Andrew Marchetti on April 29, 1954, Dr. Papanicolaou stated that the *Atlas* " is one of my last contributions to science. I thank God that I was spared long

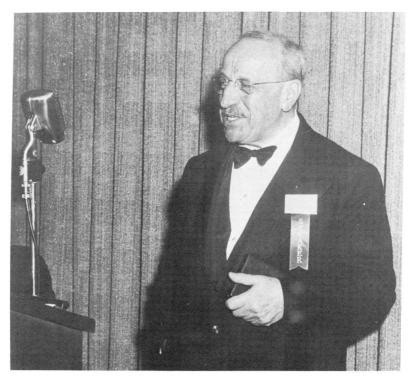

Figure 38. Dr. Papanicolaou receiving the Bertner Foundation Award in 1955, the year following his publication of the "Atlas of Exfoliative Cytology."
Please credit the University of Texas, M.D. Anderson Hospital and Tumor Clinic for the photo.

84

enough and was given the strength to complete it." Even though he continued to produce another forty-two scientific treatises, the completion of the *Atlas* ushered in a new era. Now seventy-one years old, Dr. Pap longed to reestablish closer ties with his family.

It is said that during his early years in the United States, the scientist avoided exchanging letters even with the closest members of his family. Apparently he was afraid that any communication would influence his sentiments and distract him from his work. Now with his major scientific contributions behind him, he relented somewhat in his austere approach to life and wished again to renew the close family relationships which he had enjoyed as a child. This was in part realized when a nephew and his wife bought a home in Douglaston across the street from the Papanicolaous. Their two little girls provided the enjoyment of children for their affectionate aunt and uncle. Then two nieces from Greece were alternately invited for prolonged visits. They too received the love

ATLAS OF
Exfoliative Cytology

BY GEORGE N. PAPANICOLAOU, M.D., Ph.D.
CLINICAL PROFESSOR OF ANATOMY EMERITUS. CORNELL UNIVERSITY MEDICAL COLLEGE

Published for The Commonwealth Fund by
Harvard University Press, Cambridge, Mass.
1954

Figure 39. Title page of the compendium of cytological findings in health and disease involving multiple organ systems of the human body.

CORNELL UNIVERSITY
MEDICAL COLLEGE
1300 YORK AVENUE
NEW YORK CITY

DEPARTMENT OF ANATOMY

April 29, 1954.

Dear Marchi,

Your letter has been the greatest reward I could ever receive for my Atlas. Its cordiality and warmth touched me very deeply.

I value greatly your gracious remarks about this book, which is one of my last contributions to science. I thank god that I was spared long enough and was given the strength to complete it.

I still have to add 24 more plates and I will appreciate any suggestions you may give me as to what to include in the new series. If you have any slides containing unusual cell varieties I will be very happy to add them to one of the future plates as a courteous contribution from you to my Rogue's gallery.

As I write these lines my mind goes back to the days of our joint endeavors and our thrilling adventures in a field which was then practically unexplored. I will always cherish the memory of those early pioneer days and my most pleasant association with you, which has been one of the brightest spots of my life.

Affectionately yours,
Pap

Figure 40. Letter from Dr. Papanicolaou to Dr. Andrew Marchetti during his completion of *the Atlas of Exfoliative Cytology.*

of parents from Dr. and Mrs. Papanicolaou.

Dr. Papanicolaou also began to divert some of his energy toward establishing a cytological research institute with ample space and funding to continue fundamental cell research on a broad scale. This soon became a primary objective of the still vigorous scientist. His attempts to form such an institute within the New York Hospital-Cornell Medical Center met with disappointment. Physical space was extremely limited and the establishment of an institute within an institute was contrary to policy. Dr. Pap began to look elsewhere. He had an offer from the North Shore Hospital on Long Island to set up a research laboratory. Its proximity to Douglaston, his home, made it an appealing offer, but the possible loss of continuing financial support for his work apparently influenced him to decline.

Through the years, the Papanicolaous had received invitations to return to Europe. However, the pressure of work and the tenacity with which the strict schedule was observed often prevented the couple from enjoying friends and the pleasures of

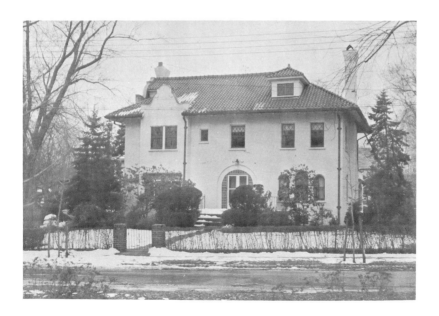

Figure 41. Second home of the Papanicolaous, Douglaston, Long Island, New York, 1957-1961.

travel. In 1957 an opportunity arose to tour Europe in conjunction with the International Cytological Congress taking place
in Brussels. A part of the tour would include a visit to Greece
where several influential citizens had urged Dr. Papanicolaou to
establish a research institute.

At the first International Cytology Conference, Dr.
Papanicolaou was made honorary president of the International
Academy of Gynecological Cytology which eventually published
the important periodical *Acta Cytologica*. Leaving Brussels, he and
Mrs. Papanicolaou visited several medical centers and friends.
Restful days were spent in Paris and the nostalgic areas along the
Cote d'Azur.

Their excitement grew as the time arrived to return to Greece.
Beginning in early August, their first stop was the Island of Corfu.
Here they were cordially received by the Greek Royal Family at
their summer home, "Mon Repos." At luncheon the possibility of
establishing a research center at the old Achelion was discussed.
The Royal Family offered this former royal residence, which now
had become a casino, to Dr. Papanicolaou, but its rather isolated
location and the uncertainty of adequate financial support led to
the abandonment of this idea. Continuing their travel through
northern Greece, they arrived in Athens in mid-August. Here Dr.
Papanicolaou met his sister and brother for the first time in
forty-four years. The family had a joyful reunion and then
proceeded to Kymi. Dr. Pap requested that no formal reception be
held for him, as he wished to spend his limited time casually
visiting old friends and landmarks.

After luncheon with his family, they visited the harbor and
walked along the beach. This must have brought back memories of
those lonesome days of frustration before his study in Germany.
The party had dinner near the sea where the nights are cool and
the atmosphere festive.

On the following day, Dr. and Mrs. Papanicolaou visited the
Cathedral of St. Athanasios and the central square where he was
greeted by a crowd of townsfolk. Later an excursion was made to
the old monastery on the hillside above the town. These were the
places he wished to see again. His last request was to visit the cap
("Kavo") by boat. When told that such a trip could be dangerous

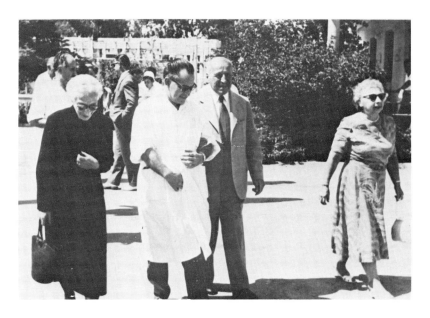

Figure 42. Dr. and Mrs. Papanicolaou, far right, visit Greece in 1957. Mrs. Nina Stamatiou, sister of Dr. Papanicolaou, is walking far left.

because of the strong wind that day, he replied, "This excursion was the goal of the whole trip for me!" He chose the largest boat in the harbor and set out with several members of his family and friends. The sea was stormy but the happy expression on the scientist's face revealed his inner satisfaction of being able to experience once again this challenging childhood feat. Past the pine-lined coast, the massive rocks of the "Kalogiros" (the priest) appeared, but the old leper colony previously there was gone. There was a moment of prayer, then the gray beaches of the cape came into view. The stormy sea caused some of the ladies to cry but the boat struggled northward until the jagged rocks of Palatia (palace) appeared. The goal had again been accomplished.

Returning to the town square, Dr. Papanicolaou was honored by the Municipal Council of Kymi and told that the central square would receive his name. Dr. Papanicolaou replied that this honor also belonged to his father who had served Kymi as mayor. Leaving the little town, only slow progress could be made because of the many well-wishers who crowded the street.

In Athens the couple maintained a busy schedule of personal appointments and meetings. There had been much discussion concerning the founding of a research center in Athens. All large hospitals and many scientists were contacted to assess the feasibility of such a project. Two wealthy Greek businessmen were involved in the discussions. However, definite decisions concerning the location and funding of such a center were not forthcoming.

After returning to New York, further correspondence about a research center in Athens did not produce encouraging results. Papanicolaou again turned his attention to the possibility of establishing a cytological research center in the United States.

In December, 1958, Dr. Papanicolaou's brother, "Nasi," died unexpectedly. He wrote his nephew-in-law, Dr. Panos Kokkoris, the following letter:

Cornell University
12/28/58

Dear Pano,

With much emotion I read your letter and I wish to thank you for the detailed narration of the disease of our dear Nasi.

The telegram of his aggravated condition disturbed us very much because it was completely unexpected. After your last letter we were waiting for clinical symptoms of his conditions.

The deep grief that I feel is mitigated only with the thought that I was able to see him even for a little while after forty-four whole years. Always I hoped that if my wish was fulfilled, I would visit Greece and I would have the pleasure of seeing him again, because when I was there I found him full of spiritual and physical vitality, in spite of all the psychic blows that he suffered in his later years. His loss will leave a huge void all around him – especially for his devoted and good partner, Petsa, and also Maria who had such exceptional love and worship for him.

Your courteous and sympathetic attendance at these trying moments is very fortunate and truly a strong support for all, especially for Maria. That's why I wish to express my gratitude for your warm brotherly concern that you have shown during these crucial hours.

Though I am far away, I feel these days of deep psychological repercussion and a vague melancholia that constantly keeps bringing recollections of our childhood under the warm roof of our father's home.

Regards from Mary and me. Good wishes for the New Year.

George.

It was shortly after this event that Dr. Papanicolaou learned that he had been proposed for the Nobel Prize in Medicine. Knowing of his nomination, it was one of his greatest disappointments to learn later that he had not been chosen. It seems that of the one hundred twenty scientists considered, only fifteen were thought to be worthy of the prize and Papanicolaou apparently ranked in third place. The unfortunate death of one of Papanicolaou's great admirers who was also a member of that Nobel Prize Committee in 1960 occurred just prior to the selection of the winner. Why Papanicolaou was not chosen is not apparent. His monumental contributions to science had received practical application on a scale rarely witnessed during one's own life. He was acknowledged as the founder of a new medical specialty.

There may have been two other factors contributing to his loss of the prize. For one, it has been said that the error of awarding the Nobel Prize in 1926 to J.A.G. Febiger for opening "a new epoch in the history of cancer,"* discouraged the awarding of the prize for a cancer discovery for 40 years. Febiger had determined twenty years before receiving the award that worms (spiroptera) rather than viruses, chemicals or irritating phenomena caused cancer. One of his countrymen later proved his work to have been in error. To be considered also is the work of Aurel Babes, alluded to earlier, which presented in the world literature almost simultaneously with Papanicolaou's first report, similar findings on uterine cancer cytology. Though disappointed that he had not been selected a Nobel laureat, he accepted the verdict calmly and continued to push his work.

The Papanicolaous' routine had not changed greatly during the years. Dr. Pap's work continued on a seven-day-a-week basis. However, more of his work was now being accomplished in the pleasant surroundings of his home. Having become Emeritus Professor of Anatomy at Cornell in 1957, he was relieved of the responsibility of being in the laboratory daily. He enjoyed spending Thursdays at home, but continued to confer with his

---

*Berland, Theodore: The Nobel Prize. *Today's Health,* Dec. 1969, p. 25.

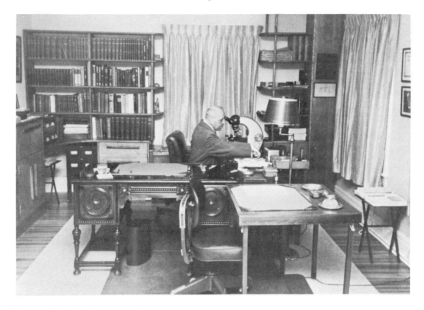

Figure 43. Dr. Papanicolaou in his study at home, Douglaston, Long Island, New York.

laboratory colleagues there. His retirement income of about six thousand dollars annually from Cornell was supplemented with a ten thousand dollar annual salary as consultant to the American Cancer Society. Too, the Papanicolaous had been frugal through the years and his modest private income from reading smears had allowed them to accumulate enough capital to live comfortably.

Mrs. Papanicolaou continued to manage all household affairs. She had the good fortune of employing a capable Japanese caretaker and cook who was with them for many years. On the weekends, Mrs. Papanicoloau herself prepared delicious Greek specialties. Her love was the garden and Dr. Pap remarked that she had "two green thumbs." But Mrs. Pap's chief concern was the welfare of her husband and she made certain that he never wanted for anything which she could provide. Cold orange juice was kept in a thermos on his desk at the laboratory and on the table beside his bed. A sandwich and fruit were brought to the office so that Dr. Pap would not have to waste time eating in the cafeteria. Mrs. Pap usually had lunch with the laboratory technicians whom she

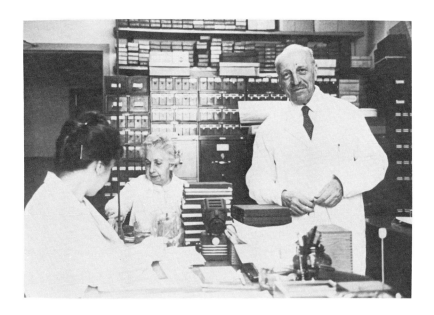

Figure 44. Dr. and Mrs. Papanicolaou in their laboratory at New York Hospital-Cornell Medical Center.

helped train. She also drove back and forth to work while Dr. Pap read or listened to the news.

On arriving home, generally after dark, the couple had dinner and then listened briefly to classical music, usually Beethoven or Bach, then Dr. Pap resumed his study until midnight or after. Their schedule on the weekends was not different from that on weekdays, except that Sunday afternoon was generally utilized for relaxation.

As plans for a cytological institute did not materialize, Papanicolaou began to turn his thoughts toward two other areas which fascinated him. These were the study of dreams and parapsychology. During his later years, he began to dream incessantly at night and he felt that many of his dreams became a reality. It was his wish to involve a psychologist who with him would launch a program to study these phenomena. Mrs. Papanicolaou was very concerned about this diversion and insisted that he maintain his scientific interest exclusively in the field of cytology.

Her hopes were vindicated when he received an offer from the Board of Directors of the Cancer Institute of Miami to become its new director. The name of the center would be changed to the Papanicolaou Cancer Research Institute. His decision to accept this offer was made without his usual consultation with his most trusted friend, Dr. Charles Cameron. Whether he felt that Dr. Cameron would oppose such a move is not known, but he invited Dr. Cameron to the "Twenty-One" for lunch and said, "I am going to Miami."

The tremendous effort required administratively to launch such an ambitious program apparently did not cause Dr. Papanicolaou to balk even though he was seventy-eight years old and unaccustomed to such problems. Because of this decision, he gave up his proposed trip to Vienna to attend the Cytological Congress held there in September 1961. There was much planning and correspondence involved in his newly assumed task.

His first task was to recruit a staff. He wrote many of his friends and former pupils. Several physicians and cytotechnologists, his photographer, Mr. Railey, and his artist came. All members of the staff had worked with Dr. Papanicolaou with the exception of Dr. Naylor. Dr. Bernard Naylor, a pathologist, would serve in addition to his other duties as liaison between the institute and other pathologists in Florida. Each member of the new staff was extremely competent in his field and had pleasing personalities. Miss Street, Dr. Papanicolaou's chief technician at Cornell, and Dr. Seybolt, his associate, remained in New York. Many found it difficult to leave their established positions and accustomed environment. Dr. Papanicolaou himself found it difficult to leave an institution which had given him opportunity, assistance and encouragement for almost half a century. He always felt a deep debt of gratitude to Cornell Medical School.

Everything was readied for moving by the end of October 1961. In early November the couple somewhat sadly departed from their home at Douglaston and moved to their comfortable new residence on DiLido Island, Miami Beach. There was much work to be done in organizing the activities of the institute. The ground floor of the institute had been completed and the diagnostic cytological laboratory preexisting in Miami had already begun work. However, the second floor, destined to be occupied by Dr. Papanicolaou and his staff, was yet unfinished. Along with solving problems at the institute, the Papanicolaous were careful to make sure that the needs of each new staff member were met. These tremendous responsibilities were accepted enthusiastically as the scientist was witnessing his last great wish come true.

Christmas 1961 was an unusually happy season for Dr. and Mrs. Papanicolaou. They were happy in their new environment and with their new "family" at the institute. In January the research laboratories began work. Dedication of the institute was scheduled to take place in May.

On Sunday, February 18, 1962, Dr. Papanicolaou spent a pleasant day with his friend, Dr. Cameron, now President of the Hahnemann Medical College and Hospital in Philadelphia, and Dr. and Mrs. Leif Jacobson of Miami. He had declined to accompany his guests on a visit to the seaquarium, but had taken his usual swim that day. Early the next morning, about 6:00 A.M., Dr. Papanicolaou suddenly noted chest pain and shortness of breath. He asked for something to drink. A physician was summoned who gave an injection for the pain. Shortly afterward he stated, "I do not feel better." These were his last words. He died shortly after arriving at Jackson Memorial Hospital. A diagnosis of coronary occlusion with heart failure and pulmonary edema was made. Mrs. Papanicolaou was unaware of any previous symptoms of coronary insufficiency, though she recalled that he occasionally had taken a pill in recent months. However, shortly after his death, one of Dr. Papanicolaou's physician friends stated that he had observed the scientist take nitroglycerine and assumed that he had angina.

Dr. Papanicolaou's body was transported to New York City, where on February 22, Archbishop Iakovos delivered a eulogy. Burial took place in New Jersey beside his beloved niece, Maria Stamatiou, herself a victim of cancer.

The remarkable life of this dedicated and gifted scientist had ended, but his contributions to the relief of suffering of his fellowman would not be forgotten. It was estimated by the American Cancer Society in 1960 that at least six million women in the United States alone had received the Pap test and that

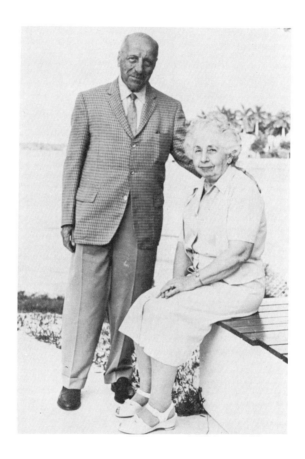

Figure 45. Dr. and Mrs. Papanicolaou at their home, DiLido Island, Miami Beach, Florida, thought to be the last photograph of Dr. Papanicolaou.

deaths from cancer of the uterus had been cut in half.

On May 13, 1962, Dr. Papanicolaou's seventy-ninth birthday, the Papanicolaou Cancer Research Institute was dedicated. In his dedication address, Dr. Cameron concluded with this summation: "He was a giver of life; he is in the company of the great; he is one of the elect of the men of earth who stand for all eternity like solitary towers along the way to human betterment. We are deeply in his debt. We rejoice that we were permitted to know him."

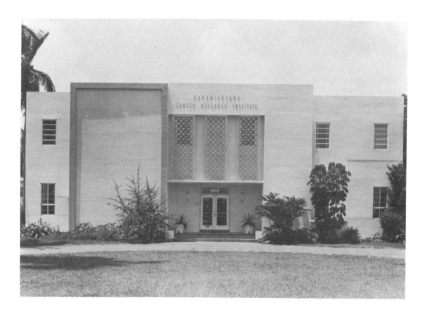

Figure 46. Papanicolaou Cancer Research Institute, Miami, Florida.

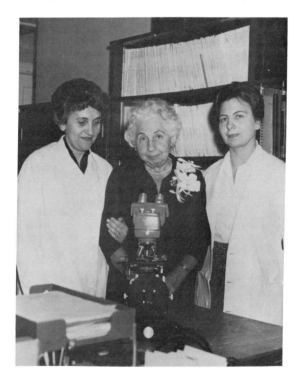

Figure 47. Mrs. Papanicolaou after receiving the American Cancer Society of Philadelphia medal for Dr. Papanicolaou posthumously.

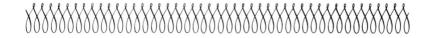

CHRONOLOGY OF EVENTS
IN THE LIFE OF
GEORGE N. PAPANICOLAOU

1883	Birth of George N. Papanicolaou.
1894-1904	To Athens for gymnasium, university and medical school.
1904-1906	Greek Army – Medical Corps.
1906-1907	Kymi (trying to convince his father to support his further education).
1907-1910	Germany – Jena, Freiburg, Munich.
1910	Married Mary Mavroyeni, to Paris, Cote d'Azur.
1911-1912	Monaco – Oceanographic Institute.
1912	Return to Germany.
1912-1913	Balkan War – Northern Greece – 1st Lt. Medical Corps.
1913	Arrived U.S.A., New York – Oct 19. Assistant in Pathology, New York Hospital.
1914-1923	Instructor in Anatomy, Cornell University (1919 – "The Existence of a Typical Oestrous Cycle in the Guinea Pig").
1923-1937	Assistant Professor of Anatomy (1928 – "New Cancer Diagnosis").
1937-1947	Associate Professor of Anatomy (1943 – "Diagnosis of Uterine Cancer by Vaginal Smear"). Professor of Anatomy (1954 – "Atlas of Exfoliative
1947-1957	Cytology"). 1948 – "Epithelia of Woman's Reproductive Tract".
1957-1961	Professor Emeritus of Anatomy (1957 – Europe revisited).
1961-1962	Director of Papanicolaou Research Institute.

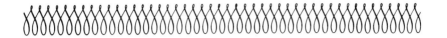

HONORS AND AWARDS

Professor Emeritus of Clinical Anatomy and Director of the Papanicolaou Research Laboratory of the Department of Anatomy, Cornell University Medical College.

Consultant to the Papanicolaou Cytology Laboratory of the Department of Pathology of the Cornell University Medical College

Consultant to the Kate Depew Strang Prevention Clinic of the Memorial Center.

Permanent Honorary Consultant to the Society of Pelvic Surgeons.

Honorary Consultant to St. Luke's Hospital, New York; North Shore Hospital, Long Island; and Perth Amboy General Hospital, New Jersey.

Member of the Medical Advisory Board, Medico.

Member of the New York City Department of Health, Cancer Advisory Committee.

Honorary Member of the American Society for the Study of Sterility.

Honorary Member of the Obstetrical and Gynecological Society of Athens.

Honorary Member of the Obstetrical-Gynecological Society of Buenos Aires.

Honorary Member of the First Argentine Congress on Cancer (1952).

Honorary Member of the New York Academy of Sciences; American Association for the Advancement of Science and the First Honorary Member of the Academy of Athens.

Honorary Fellowship, American College of Clinical Pathologists, 1956.

Honorary Fellowship, International College of Surgeons, 1956
Honorary Member of the James Ewing Society (1958)
Awarded Honorary Degrees by the University of Athens,
Greece; University of Turin, Italy; and the Hahnemann Medical
College of Philadelphia.
Borden Award, Association of American Medical College, 1948.
Amory Award, American Association of Arts and Sciences,
1948.
Lasker Award, American Public Health Association, 1950.
First Award of the Order of AHEPA, as the Most Outstanding
American Scientist of Greek Descent, 1951.
The Honor Medal of the American Cancer Society, 1952.
The Wien Award for Exfoliative Cytology, 1953.
The Cross of the Grand Commander of Royal Order of Phoenix,
presented by the King of Greece in December of 1953.
The Modern Medicine Award for Distinguished Achievement,
1954.
The Bertner Award, 1955.
The Passano Award, 1956.
Honorary Award, German Gynecological Society, 1956.
Honorary Award, Virginia Division of The American Cancer
Society, 1956.
Alvarenga Prize, 1957.
Century Award, General Federation of Women's Clubs, 1957.
Gold Medal, Greek Red Cross, 1957.
Royal Order of George the First, presented by the Greek
Government in April of 1957.
Honorary Award, Brazilian Cytology Society, 1957.
Clement Cleveland Award, 1960.

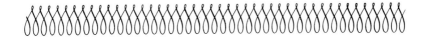

SOURCES OF AUTHOR'S MATERIAL

Most of my information has been assimilated from personal interviews. However, certain historical background material and biographical documentation were acquired from existing publications.

For the history of Kymi, I relied principally on a short Greek tract entitled "Kymi – Balcony of the Aegean," by Nicholas X. Karapas. Dr. Richard Goldschmidt in his two delightful books, *In and Out of the Ivory Tower* and *Portraits From Memory, Recollections of a Zoologist,* provided an excellent description of life in Munich and the Hertwig Institute during the years Dr. Papanicolaou was there.

A better understanding of the oceanographic cruises of Prince Albert I was obtained from "Resultats des campagnes scientifiques accomplies sur son yacht," by Albert I, Prince of Monaco (*Fascicule* 89-1934) and *Bulletin De L'Institut Oceanographique* (No. 234, June 12, 1912). For details of the rather politically complicated Balkan War, I utilized Schurman's *The Balkan Wars 1912-1913.*

Since minor descrepancies occasionally were noted in the many memorial articles which were published shortly after Dr. Papanicolaou's death, I have depended primarily on Dr. Papanicolaou's own publications, those of Dr. Charles Cameron and in addition, two interviews, as sources of previously published biographical data. One interview was conducted and edited by Frederick Flach for the *Cornell Medical Journal,* December 1948. "A Visit with Dr. George N. Papanicolaou," derived from an interview by Dr. Samuel Berkow, appeared in the journal, *Obstetrics and Gynecology,* August 1960.

Much of the history of endocrine cytology was selected from two of Dr. George Corner's publications. One entitled, "The Early History of the Oestrogenic Hormones," was delivered in Middlesex Hospital, London, as the Sir Henry Dale lecture for 1964. The other, a book, *The Hormones in Human Reproduction,* was published in 1947.

The anecdotal information concerning the Woman's Hospital in New York was found in Dr. James P. Marr's "J. Marion Sims,"1957, and "That Many May Live" by Bob Considine (Memorial Center for Cancer and Allied Diseases 1959).

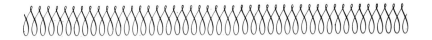

LIST OF PUBLICATIONS BY
GEORGE N. PAPANICOLAOU, M.D., PH.D.

1. **1910.** Uber die Bedingungen der sexuellen Differenzierung bei Daphniden. *Biologisches Centralblatt,* B. 30.
2. **1910.** Experimentelle Untersuchungen uber die Fortpflanzungsverhaltnisse der Daphniden. *Biologisches Centralblatt,* B. 30.
3. **1915.** Sex determination and sex control in guinea-pigs. *Science, 41:*401.
4. **1916.** A further analysis of the hereditary transmission of degeneracy and deformities by the descendants of alcoholized mammals. II. *American Naturalist, 50* (Stockard, Charles R. and Papanicolaou, George N.).
5. **1916.** American Assoc. Anat — Specimens illustrating the histology of proestrous and ovulation guinea-pig. (Proceedings of American Assoc. Anat., Dec. 1916, p. 128).
6. **1916.** Microscopic preparations showing various stages in the developmental changes of the idiosome. (Demonstration American Assoc. Anat., Dec. 1916, p. 127).
7. **1917.** A rhythmical "heat period" in the guinea-pig. *Science, 46:*1176:42-44 Stockard, C. R. and Papanicolaou, G. N.).
8. **1917.** The existence of a typical oestrous cycle in the guinea-pig — with a study of its histological and physiological changes. *Am J Anat, 22:*2:225-283; 1917 (Stockard, C. R. and Papanicolaou, G.N.).
9. **1918.** The development of the idiosome in the germ-cells of the male guinea-pig. *Am J Anat, 24:*1 (Papanicolaou, George N. and Stockard, Charles R.).
10. **1918.** Further studies on the modification of the germ-cells in mammals: The effect of alcohol on treated guinea-pigs and their descendants. *J Exp Zool, 26:*1 (Stockard, Charles R. and Papanicolaou, George N.).
11. **1919.** The vaginal closure membrane, copulation and the vaginal plug in the guinea-pig, with further considerations of the oestrous rhythm. *Biol Bull, 37:*3 (Stockard, Charles R. and Papanicolaou, George N.).

12. **1920.** Influence of removal of corpora lutea and ripe follicles on the oestrous periodicity in guinea-pig. *Anatomical Record, 18:*32;1920.

13. **1920.** Effect of underfeeding on ovulation and the oestrous rhythm in guinea-pigs. *Proc Soc Exp Biol Med,* 107th Meeting (Papanicolaou, George N. and Stockard, Charles R.).

14. **1921.** Developmental competition in its relationship to the sex ratio. *Anatomical Record,* March, 1921, p. 36.

15. **1922.** Morphology of cystic growths in the ovary and uterus of the guinea pig. *Pro Soc Exp Bio Med, 19:*401-402. (Papanicolaou, George N. and Stockard, C. R.).

16. **1922.** Experimental results bearing on the etiology of cystic growths in the ovary and uterus of the guinea-pig. *Pro Soc Exp Bio Med,* 402-403 (Papanicolaou, G. N. and Stockard, C. R.).

17. **1923.** The ovarian cystic fluid with special reference to its effect upon the reactions of the genital tract. *Pro Soc Exp Bio Med, 21:*164-166 (Papanicolaou, G.N. and Blau, N.F.).

18. **1923.** Oestrus in mammals from a comparative point of view. *Am J Anat, 32:*3;1923.

19. **1924.** Ovogenesis during sexual maturity as elucidated by experimental methods. *Pro Soc Exp Biol Med, 21:*393-396.

20. **1924.** The production of certain distinct types of reactions by the use of ovarian extracts. *Proc Soc Exp Biol Med, 22:*106-108.

21. **1925.** The diagnosis of early human pregnancy by the vaginal smear method. *Proc Soc Exp Biol Med, 22:*436-437.

22. **1926.** A specific inhibitory hormone of the corpus luteum. Its contrast with the female sex (follicular) hormone. JAMA, 86.

23. **1927.** A case of hermaphroditismus verus lateralis in a guinea-pig. *Anat Rec, 36:*3; Sept. 25 (Jaffe, Henry and Papanicolaou, George N.).

24. **1927.** The mechanism of the periodical opening and closing of the vaginal orifice in the guinea-pig. *Am J Anat, 40:*2; Nov. 15 (Kelly, George Lombard and Papanicolaou, George N.).

25. **1927.** Existence of a sexual rhythm and experimental induction of heat in the dog during anoestrus. *Anat Rec, 35:*47 (Papanicolaou, G. N. and Blau, N. F.).

26. **1928.** New cancer diagnosis. Proc. Third Race Betterment Con., 528.

27. **1928.** Monocytic reactions in the vagina. *Anat Rec, 38:*55-56; 1928.

28. **1929.** Ovulation in man and mammals. *NY State J Med,* p. 1.

29. **1931.** Specificity of reactions produced by injection of urine from pregnant cows into immature female guinea pigs. *Proc Soc Exp Biol Med, 28:*807.

30. **1931.** Specific adrenal reactions as induced by injections of urine from pregnant cows and women. *Anat Rec,* Feb., 1931, p. 59.

31. **1932.** Observations on the periodic replacement of the uterine

epithelium in the guinea-pig. *Anat Rec,* Feb., 1932, p. 29.

32. **1933.** Epithelial regeneration in the uterine glands and on the surface of the uterus. *Am J Obstet Gynecol, 25:*1,30.

33. **1933.** The sexual cycle in the human female as revealed by vaginal smear. *Am J Anat 52:*3;519-637 (supplement) May.

34. **1933.** The existence of a "postmenopause" sexual rhythm in women, as indicated by the study of vaginal smears. *Anat Rec, 55:*71.

35. **1933.** The modifying effect of old age upon the oestrous cycle in the guinea-pig. *Anat Rec, 55:*71.

36. **1934.** Action of pregnancy urine extract (follutein) on the external genitalia of female guinea pigs. *Proc Soc Exp Biol Med, 31:*750-751 (Papanicoloau, George N., and Falk, Emil A.).

37. **1935.** Action of ovarian follicle hormone in ovarian insufficiency in women as indicated by vaginal smears. *Proc Soc Exp Biol Med, 32:*585-587 (Papanicolaou, George N. and Shorr, Ephraim).

38. **1936.** On the continuation of sexual rhythms in a woman after menopause. Am. Assoc. Anat. abstract copied from *Anat Rec, 64:*37.

39. **1936.** Effect of pregnancy urine extract (follutein) upon normal and transplanted gonads and upon the external genitalia in guinea pigs. *Anat Rec, 64* (Falk, Emil A., and Papanicolaou, George N.).

40. **1936.** The action of ovarian follicular hormone in the menopause as indicated by vaginal smears. *Am J Obstet Gynecol, 31:*5,806 (Papanicolaou, George N. and Shorr, Ephraim).

41. **1937.** Differences in the reactions of normal and transplanted ovaries in guinea-pigs, to pregnancy urine hormone (follutein). *Anat Rec, 67:*38;1937 (Papanicolaou, George N. and Falk, Emil A.).

42. **1938.** Inhibitory effects of male sex hormone in human menstruation and their evaluation by vaginal smears. *Proc Soc Exp Biol Med, 37:*689-692 (Papanicolaou, George N.; Ripley, Herbert S. and Shorr, Ephraim).

43. **1938.** General muscular hypertrophy induced by androgenic hormone. *Science, 87:*2254:238-239 (Papanicolaou, George N. and Falk, Emil A.).

44. **1938.** Growth, desquamation and involution of the vaginal epithelium of fetuses and children with a consideration of the related hormonal factors. *Am J Anat, 62:*4;May 15 (Fraenkel, Ludwig and Papanicolaou, George Nicholas).

45. **1938.** The production of general muscular hypertrophy by the androgenic hormone. *Anat Rec 70:*4:61 (supplement no. 3) (Papanicolaou, George N. and Falk, Emil A.).

46. **1938.** The effect of sympathectomy upon the sex functions of female guinea-pigs. *Anat Rec 70:*4:62 (supplement no. 3) (Phillips, R. A. and Papanicolaou, G. N.)

47. **1938.** Neutralization of ovarian follicular hormone in women by simultaneous administration of male sex hormone. *Proc Soc Exp Biol Med, 38:*759-762 (Shorr, Ephraim; Papanicolaou, George N.; Stimmel, Benjamin F.).

48. **1938.** The effect of androgenic hormone on activity in male and female guinea-pigs. 46th Meeting of the American Psychological Association, *Abstracts,* Sept., 1938, p. 44 (Seward, John P., Papanicolaou, George N.).

49. **1939.** Suppressive action of testosterone propionate on menstruation and its effect on vaginal smears. *Endocrinology, 24:*3:339-346 (Papanicolaou, George N.; Ripley, Herbert S.; Shorr, Ephraim).

50. **1939.** Sex functions in the senile female guinea-pig. *Anat Rec, 73:*(no. 3, supplement no. 2): 40-41.

51. **1939.** Action of gonadotropic hormones in amenorrhea as evaluated by vaginal smears. *Proc Soc Exp Biol Med, 41:*629-636 (Shorr, Ephraim and Papanicolaou, George N.).

52. **1939.** Artificial oestrus in the guinea-pig without ovaries and uterus. *Psychol Bull, 36:*7 (Papanicolaou, George N. and Seward, John P.).

53. **1939.** The relation of estrogen therapy in the human carcinogenesis. Third International Cancer Congress, Atlantic City, 9/11-9/15, 1939, p. 90. (Shorr, Ephraim and Papanicolaou, George N.)

54. **1939.** A clinical study of the synthetic estrogen stilbestrol. *JAMA, 113:*2312-2318 (Shorr, Ephraim; Robinson, Frank; Papanicolaou, George N.).

55. **1940.** The effect of treatment of depression in the menopause with estrogenic hormone. *Am J Psychiatry, 96:*4 (Ripley, Herbert S.; Shorr, Ephraim; Papanicolaou, George N.)

56. **1941.** Periodic activation of the histiocytes in the vaginal fluid. *Anat Rec, 79:*(no. 3):75-76.

57. **1941.** Menstrual cycle with vaginal smear studies in schizophrenia, depression, and elation. Abstract, presented by Dr Ripley at the Annual Meeting of Psychiatric Assoc., May 18, 1941.

58. **1940.** Studies of spontaneous tumors in guinea-pigs. I. A. fibromyoma of the stomach with adenoma (focal hyperplasia) of the right adrenal. *Am J Cancer 40:*3;1940 (Papanicolaou, George N. and Olcott, Charles T.).

59. **1941.** The diagnostic value of vaginal smears in carcinoma of the uterus. *Am J Obstet Gynecol, 42:*2:193-206. (Papanicolaou, G. N. and Traut, H. F.).

60. **1942.** Vaginal smear changes in endometrial hyperplasias and in cervical keratosis. *Anat Rec, 82* (Traut, Herbert F. and Papanicolaou, George N.).

61. **1942.** Cancer cells in vaginal smears. *Anat Rec, 82* (Papanicolaou, George N. and Traut, Herbert F.).

62. **1942.** The demonstration of malignant cells in vaginal smears and its relation to the diagnosis of carcinoma of the uterus. *N Y State J Med, 43:*8;1943 (Papanicolaou, G. N. and Traut, H. F.).

63. **1942.** The menstrual cycle with vaginal smear studies in schizophrenia, depression and elation. *Am J Psychiatry, 98:*4 (Ripley, Herbert S. and Papanicolaou, George N.).

64. **1942.** A new procedure for staining vaginal smears. *Science, 95:*2469:438-439; 1942.

65. **1942.** Studies of spontaneous tumors in guinea-pigs. II. Tumors of the stomach and intestine. *Arch Pathol, 34* 218-228 (Papanicolaou, George N. and Olcott, Charles T.).

66. **1943.** Studies on spontaneous tumors in guinea-pigs. III. A chondrosarcoma of the iliac bone with metastasis to the mammary region. *Cancer Research 3:*5; 1943 (Olcott, Charles T. and Papanicolaou, George N.).

67. **1943.** Diagnosis of Uterine Cancer by the Vaginal Smear. The Commonwealth Fund, New York, N. Y., May, 1943 (Papanicolaou, George N. and Traut, Herbert F.).

68. **1943.** Cancer of the uterus: The vaginal smear in its diagnosis. *California and Western Medicine, 59:*2;1943 (Traut, Herbert F. and Papanicolaou, George N.).

69. **1943.** The use of endocervical and endometrial smears in the diagnosis of cancer and of other conditions of the uterus. *Am J Obstet Gynecol, 46:*3:421-422;1943 (Papanicolaou, G. N. and Marchetti, A. A.).

70. **1944.** El frotis dela secrecion vaginal como metodo de diagnostico del cancer del utero. *Am Clin 7:*5-6:109-115; 1944.

71. **1945.** Some characteristic changes in the consistency of the uterine secretion. *Anat rec, 91:*4:31.

72. **1945.** Urine sediment smears as a diagnostic procedure in cancers of the urinary tract. *Science, 101:*2629:519-520 (Papanicolaou, George N. and Marshall, Victor F.).

73. **1945.** The vaginal and endometrial smear as a diagnostic procedure in cancer of the uterus. *N Y State J Med, 45:*12:1336;1945.

74. **1946.** A general survey of the vaginal smear and its use in research and diagnosis. *Am J Obstet Gynecol, 51:*3:316-324;1946.

75. **1946.** Diagnostic value of exfoliated cells from cancerous tissues. *JAMA, 131:*372-378;1946.

76. **1947.** Cytology of the urine sediment in endoplasms of the urinary tract. *J Urol, 57:*2;1947.

77. **1947.** The cytology of the gastric fluid in the diagnosis of carcinoma of the stomach. *J. Natl Cancer Inst, 7:*5:537;1947 (Papanicolaou, George N.; Cooper, William A.).

78. **1948.** The cell smear method of diagnosing cancer. *Am J Public Health, 38:*2;1948.

79. **1948.** Diagnosis of pregnancy by cytologic criteria in catheterizer urine. *Proc Soc Exp Biol Med, 67:*247-249,1948.

80. **1948.** The Epithelia of Woman's productive organs. The Commonwealth Fund, N. Y. March, 1948 (Papanicolaou, George N.; Traut, Herbert F.; Marchetti, Andrew A.).

81. **1948.** The cell smear method of diagnosing cancer. Proc. New York State Assoc. Public Health Lab. 27:2:60-66.

82. **1948.** The diagnosis of cancer by cytologic criteria. Proc. New York Path. Soc., April 24, 1947.

83. **1949.** Early renal carcinoma *in situ.* Detected by means of smears of fixed urinary sediment. *JAMA, 139:*356-358 (Foot, N. Chandler and Papanicolaou, G. N.).

84. **1949.** Cytology of bronchial secretions. *J Thorac Cardiovasc Surg 18:*1:113-122; 1949.

85. **1941.** Diagnosis of cancer of the lung by the cytologic method. *Diseases of the Chest, 15:*4:412;1949 (Papanicolaou, George N. and Cromwell, Henry A.).

86. **1949.** Cytologic diagnosis of uterine cancer by examination of vaginal and uterine secretions. *Am J Clin Pathol, 19:*4:301-308;1949.

87. **1949.** A survey of the actualities and potentialities of exfoliative cytology in cancer diagnosis. *Ann Intern Med, 31:*4;1949.

88. **1950.** Abrasive ballon for exfoliation of gastric cancer cells. *JAMA, 143:*1308-1311;1950 (Panico, Frederick G.; Papanicolaou, George N. and Cooper, William A.).

89. **1951.** Cytology in the diagnosis of gastric cancer. *Cancer, 4:*2;1951 (Seybolt, John F. and Papanicolaou, George N.; Cooper, William A.).

90. **1951.** Cytologic diagnosis of gastric cancer. A chapter in Pack and McNeer's book *Gastric Cancer* (Papanicolaou, G. N. and Seybolt, John F.).

91. **1951.** Carcinoma *in situ* of the right lower bronchus. A case report. *Cancer, 4:*1;1951 (Papanicolaou, George N. and Koprowska, Irene).

92. **1951.** The examination of exfoliated cells in tumor diagnosis. A chapter for the second edition of *Treatment of Cancer and Allied Diseases,* edited by George T. Pack and Irving M. Ariel. (Papanicolaou, George N. and Foot, N. C.).

93. **1952.** The application of cytology in the diagnosis of cancer of the rectum, sigmoid, and descending colon. *Cancer, 5:*2:307-314;1952 (Bader, Genevieve M. and Papanicolaou, George N.).

94. **1951.** Criteria for the diagnosis of malignancy by smear methods. At the Symposium of Exfoliated Cytology, Annual Meeting of the American Cancer Society, Oct., 1951.

95. **1951.** Value of gastric smears in early diagnosis of gastric cancer.

Presented at the Symposium of Exfoliated Cytology, Annual Meeting of the American Cancer Society, Oct., 1951.

96. **1953.** Recent trends in cytologic diagnosis. *N Y State J Med, 53:*1; 1953.

97. **1953.** Use of the cytologic method in industrial medicine. *A M A Archives of Industrial Hygiene and Occupational Medicine, 5:*3:232-233;1952.

98. **1952.** Present status and future trends of exfoliative cytology. Ca.-Bull. of Cancer Progress 2:50-56, March, 1952.

99. **1952.** The balloon techniques in the detection of gastric carcinoma. Proc. of the Second National Cancer Conference, 1952 (Seybolt, John F. and Papanicolaou, George N.).

100. **1952.** Cytologic examination of breast secretions. Proc. of the Second National Cancer Conference.

101. **1952,** Observations on the origin of histiocytes in secretions of the female genital tract. *Anat Rec 112:*69;1952.

102. **1952.** A microfluorometric scanning method for the detection of cancer cells in smears of exfoliated cells. *Cancer, 5:*3;1952 (Mellors, Robert C.; Glassman, Adele; Papanicolaou, George N.).

103. **1952.** Nucleic acid content of the squamous cancer cell. *Science, 116:*3011:265-269; 1952.

104. **1953.** Balloon technique in the cytological diagnosis of gastric cancer. *JAMA, 151:*10-14; 1953 (Cooper, William A. and Papanicolaou, George N.).

105. **1951.** Evaluation of mitosis in smears. Presented at Symposium on Exfoliative Cytology, Annual Meeting of the American Cancer Society, Oct., 1951.

106. **1953.** Exfoliative cytology. Chapter in a book *Cancer of the Lung* by Rosenblatt, et al. (Foot, N. C. and Papanicolaou, George N.).

107. **1953.** Observations on the origin and specific function of the histiocytes in the female genital tract. *Fertil Steril, 4:*6;1953.

108. **1952.** The detection of early cancer, Panel Discussion of 32nd Practitioner's Conference, New York Hospital, Jan. 30, 1952. (reprinted in N.Y.H.).

109. **1954.** Cytologic studies in diagnosis of carcinoma. *J Int Coll Surg 21:*4:419-426;1954.

110. **1954.** Exfoliative cytology in carcinoma of the cervix. American Medical Convention, Carcinoma of the cervix. June, 1953, New York City.

111. **1953.** Cytologic examination of breast secretions. Proc. of the Second Nat. Cancer Conference. (Discussion in paper by Dr. Otto Saphir).

112. **1954.** La citologia nello studio e nella diagnosi del cancro dell'utero. *Minerva Ginecologica, 6:*9;1954.

113. **1953.** Citologia Exfoliativa: Su valor en el diagnostico del cancer. (Exfoliative cytology: Its value in the diagnosis of cancer.) *Arch Med Cuba 4:*579-586;1953 (Seybolt, J. F. and Papanicolaou, George N.).

114. **1954.** Cytological evaluation of smears prepared by the tampon method for the detection of carcinoma of the uterine cervix. *Cancer, 7:*6:1185-1190;1954.

115. **1954.** The value of exfoliative cytology in the diagnosis and control of neoplastic disease of the breast. *California Bulletin of Cancer Progress, 4:*6:191-197;1954.

116. **1954.** *Atlas of Exfoliative Cytology.* Published for the Commonwealth Fund by Harvard University Press, Cambridge, Mass.

117. **1955.** Cytology of esophageal washings. Evaluation of 364 cases. *Cancer, 8:*5;1955 (Johnson, William D.; Koss, Leopold G.; Papanicolaou, George N.; Seybolt, John F.).

118. **1955.** Vaginal cytology in trichomonas infestation. *International Record of Medical and General Practice Clinics, 168:*9;1955 (Papanicolaou, George N.; Wolinska, Wanda H.).

119. **1955.** The evolutionary dynamics and trends of exfoliative cytology. *Texas Report on Biology and Medicine, 13:*4:901-919;1955.

120. **1955.** Appraisal of the diagnostic value of the endometrial aspiration smear. Proc. Scientific Sessions of the Am. Can. Soc.

121. **1956.** Cytologic evaluation of breast secretions. *Annals of the New York Academy of Sciences, 63:*6:1409-1421 (Papanicolaou, George N.; Bader, Genevieve M.; Holmquist, Doris G.; Falk, Emil A.).

122. **1956.** The exfoliative cytology of the mammary gland during pregnancy and lactation. *Annals of the New York Academy of Sciences, 63:*6:1422-1435;1956 (Holmquist, Doris G.; Papanicolaou, George N.).

123. **1956.** Supplement No. 1 of the *Atlas of Exfoliative Cytology.* Published for the Commonwealth Fund by Harvard University Press, Cambridge, Mass., 1956.

124. **1956.** Degenerative changes in ciliated cells exfoliating from the bronchial epithelium as a cytologic criterion in the diagnosis of diseases of the lung. *N Y State J Med, 56:*17;1956.

125. **1956.** Exfoliative cytologic patterns in carcinoma *in situ* correlated with histopathologic findings. Proc. Third Nat. Cancer Conference.

126. **1956.** Exfoliative cytology in research and diagnosis. (read at the AMA meeting on the occasion of the presentation of the Passano Award, June,1956.) California Bulletin of Cancer Progress, 6:*(no. 6):1956.

127. **1957.** Detection of endometrial adenocarcinoma by tampon-smear method. *Cancer, 10:*1;1957 (Brunschwig, Alexander;

Papanicolaou, George N.).
128. **1957.** The cancer – diagnostic potential of uterine exfoliative cytology. *Cancer Bulletin, 7:*4;1957.
129. **1957.** Simple method for protecting fresh smears from drying and deterioration during mailing. *JAMA, 164:*1957 (Papanicolaou, George N.; Bridges, Emma Lou).
130. **1955,** Cytologic changes simulating those of cancer. (read at I.S.C.C. meeting in Clevland, Nov., 1955.).
131. **1955.** On the morphologic relationship of duct epithelial cells and foam cells as observed in breast secretion smears. (read by title at I.S.C.C. meeting in Clevland, Nov., 1955).
132. **1956.** Historical landmarks in exfoliative cytology. Proc. of the International Cancer Cytology Congress, Chicago, 1956.
133. **1956.** Personnel in Cytology. Proc. of the International Cancer Cytology Congress, Chicago, 1956.
134. **1957.** Investigative and diagnostic aspects of exfoliative cytology. Trans. of the College of Physicians of Philadelphia 4 Wer., *25:* (no.2):1957.
135. **1957.** The actual value of cytology in the diagnosis of upper gastro – intestinal malignancies, V Congreso Pan Am. de Gastroenterologia, Tomo 1, Memoria, 304-314 (Seybolt, J. F. and Papanicolaou, G. N.).
136. **1957.** Exfoliative cytology of the human mammary gland and its value in the diagnosis of cancer and other diseases of the breast. *Cancer, 11:*2:377-409;1958. (Papanicoloau, G. N.; Holmquist, D. G.; Gader, G. M.; Falk, V. A.).
137. **1957.** Cellular changes in the development of pulmonary cancer as revealed by the Cytology: A case report. *Acta Union International Contre le Cancer, 14:*4:479-84;1958.
138. **1957.** Historical development of cytology as a tool in clinical medicine and in cancer research. *Acta International Contre le Cancer, 14:*4:249-54, 1958.
139. **1957.** Observations on the behavior of endometrial cells in tissue culture. *Am J Obstet Gynecol, 76:*3:601-18;1958 (Papanicolaou, G. N. and Maddi, Frances V.).
140. **1957.** The value of cytology in the diagnosis of gastric cancer. *Gastroenterology, 33:*3:369-77;1957 (Seybolt, J. F. and Papanicolaou, G. N.).
141. **1957.** Further observations on the behavior of human endometrial cells *in virto. Am J Obstet Gynecol, 78:*1:156-173;1959 (Papanicolaou, G. N. and Maddi, F. V.).
142. **1958.** The diagnosis of pancreatic cancer by cytologic study of duodenal secretions. *Acta Union International Contre le Cancer, 16:*(no. 2):398-404;1960 (Bowden, Lemuel and **Papanicolaou,** G. N.).

143. **1958.** Exfoliated pancreatic cancer cells in the duct of wirsung. *Ann Surg, 150:*2:296-98;1959 (Bowden, K. and Papanicolaou, G. N.).

144. **1959.** Significance of exfoliative cytology in gynecological research and diagnosis. (Joint meeting Jan. 1959 of Buffalo Acad. of Med. & Buffalo Ob. & Gyn. Soc.).

145. **1959.** Endometrial Cytology (Feb. 1959, Hahnemann Med. Coll., Cytology, Lab.).

146. **1959.** Pitfalls in exfoliative cytology. (Path. Institute, Johns Hopkins).

147. **1959.** Exfoliative cytology and its value to the general practitioner. (Suffolk County Chapter, A. of G.P.).

148. **1959.** Cytology in relation to pelvic physiology and/or disease. 31st annual Stuart McGuire Lecture Series, Society of Pelvic Surgeons, Med. Coll. of Virginia.

149. **1959.** Introduction to symposium on dyskaryosis. *Acta Cytol, 1:*1;1957.

150. **1960.** Statement prepared for science writers' seminar. American Cancer Society, Louisville Meeting. G. N. Papanicolaou – read by Cynthia Pierce, 3/37/60. March.

151. **1960.** Chapter on Exfoliative Cytology. SYMPOSIUM ON CANCER. *Modern Medicine, 28:*7:89-96;1960 (G. N. Papanicolaou).

152. **1960.** Supplement No. 2 of the *Atlas of Exfoliative Cytology.*

153. **1960.** Diagnostic value of cells of endometrial and ovarian origin in human tissue cultures. *Acta Cytol, 5:*1:1961 (Papanicolaou, G. N. and Maddi, F. V.).

154. **1960.** Degeneration of the ciliated cells of the bronchial epithelium (Ciliocytophthoria) in its relation to pulmonary disease. *Am Rev Resp Dis,* 1961 (Papanicolaou, G. N.; Bridges, E.; Railey, C. J.).

155. **1960.** The role of exfoliative cytology in diagnosis and research. Read before the Queen's Division of the American Cancer Society, Nov. 29, 1960.

156. **1960.** Memorandum on Staining. (Prepared for distribution with Supplement No.2).

157. **1961.** Dramatic news in uterine cancer. General Federation *Clubwoman,* 8;1961.

158. **1961.** Diagnostic significance of ciliated cells in human endometrial tissue cultures. *Am J Obstet Gynecol,* 99;1961 (Maddi, F. V. and Papanicolaou, G. N.).

INDEX

O

Ovarian estrogenic hormone, detection
of, 51
Ovulation period determination, guinea
pigs,
Papanicolaou study, 47-48

P

"Pap" smear, mass testing, 83
see also Smear technique, and Vaginal
smears
Papaevangelos, Maria, xv
Papajohn, Steve, xvi
Papanicolaou, Athanase, grandfather of
George, 6
Papanicolaou, George Nicholas,
abnormal conditions studied by
smears, 62
Athens,
early experiences, 10-11
offer from university, 52
visits brother and sister, 88
amenorrheic women studied, 63
Atlantis paper assignment, 45
"Atlas of Exfoliative Cytology,"
completed in 1954, 83
comments on, 84-85
awards and honors, 101-102
Balkan war service, 41-43
biography, chronology, events in his
life, 99
biological research interest roused, 19
birth, childhood, and early education,
viii-ix, xi, 6-7
bowlegs corrected, 17
boyhood self-discipline, viii, xi
brother "Nasi" dies, 90-91
cancer cell studies, 74
cautions against premature publicity,
76
cell staining technique development,
65
character, viii
childhood, xi, 3-9
chronology of events in his life, 99
clinical use of vaginal smear
recognized, 54

comments on cool reception of paper
on cancer studies, 60-61
Commonwealth Fund, 1941 grant, 71
confidence in conclusions, given by
1942 cases, 72
Cornell Medical School,
appointment, 45
becomes Emeritus Professor of
Anatomy in 1957, 91
cytological research aided, 65-66
daphnia sex studies, 23
death Feb. 18, 1962, 95
description by Munich associates,
23-25
"Diagnosis of Uterine Cancer by Vaginal Smear," 1943 monograph,
73
diagnostic potentialities of vaginal
smear investigated, 62-63
"Diagnostic Value of Vaginal Smears
in Carcinoma of the Uterus,"
1941 paper, 69-70
Douglaston home, move to, 66
early personality, 6
early political interests, 9
education, 10-17
"Epithelia of Woman's Reproductive
Organs," 78-83
"Epithelia of Woman's Reproductive
Organs," 1948 monograph, 76
estrogenic compounds studied, 65
estrous cycle studies, 47-49
ethinyl estradiol, stilbestrol compared,
65
exercise schedule, xii
family enjoyments, 85-87
father,
death, 52
selection of wife for son, 27
first American publication, 1915, 47
first observation of cancer cells in
smear, 56
first paper on human vaginal smears,
56
funeral in New York, burial in New
Jersey, 95
German philosophy influence, xi
Germany, studies in Jena, 17
Gimbel's department store work, 45

Gimbel's department store work, 45
home life, gardening, Japanese caretaker and cook, 92-93
"special" case in husband's studies, 54
wife of Dr. Papanicolaou, ix
see also Mavroyeni
Papanicolaou, Nicholas,
education, 6
father of George N., 6
characteristics as parent, 9
married life, 6
objection to George going to America, 43
selection of wife for George, 27
Papanicolaou Cancer Research Center,
dedication, 96
Papanicolaou made director, 94
Papanicolaou test, vii
see also "Pap" smear
Pathological cases, vaginal smear studies, 56
Pathological changes, Papanicolaou's studies of smears, 62
Physalia jelly fish, studies, 29
Portier, jellyfish studies, 29
Potter, Henry, looks toward disease prevention, 60
Pouchet, human vaginal smears described, 54
Pregnancy, diagnosis by vaginal smear, 56
Prince Albert I of Monaco,
oceanographic research interest, 29
oceanographic expedition, daily schedule, 34-36
Prohibition, alcohol's influence of interest, 47
Prostate secretions, cancer detection, 78
Psychiatric patients, vaginal smear studies, 65
Publications by Papanicolaou, 105-115

R

Railey, Papanicolaou's photographer, 94
Ray, L. Beatrice, xvi
Religious philosophy, Ernst Haeckel, 18-19

Richard, on oceanographic expedition, 34
Richet, jellyfish studies, 29
Riddle of the Universe, Haeckel's defense of philosophy, 19
Rust, Dominique, xv

S

St. Athanasios Basilica, in Kymi square, 4, 6
Schleiden, botanical discovery, 18
Schwann, Theodor, cell structure demonstration, 18
Shorr, Ephraim,
discontinues work with Papanicolaou, 68
modification of cell staining technique, 65
1934 studies with Papanicolaou, 63
Science, 19th century advances, 18
Science,
animal smear studies article by Papanicolaou, 49
"Sex Determination . . . ," by Papanicolaou, 47
Sepsas, Maria, xv
"Sex Determination and Sex Control in Guinea Pigs,"
article by Papanicolaou, 47
"The Sexual Cycle of the Human Female," paper by Papanicolaou, 63
Seybolt, Papanicolaou's associate, 94
Sims, Marion,
founder of Woman's Hospital, 57-60
stand on aid to cancer patients, 57-60
Smear technique, cancers in various areas detected, 76-78
see also "Pap" smear, and Vaginal smears
Spinal fluid, cancer detection, 78
Sputum, cancer detection, 78
Stamatiou, Nina, xv
Stander, H. J., supports Papanicolaou's cancer detection studies, 68-69
Stangpwitz, friend of Papanicolaou, 40